7

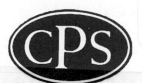

**This book is to be returned on or before
the last date stamped below.**

LIBREX

7/10   RJ

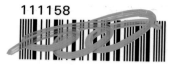

THE AUTHOR

HARRIET SERGEANT is the author of the widely-acclaimed *Welcome to the Asylum: immigration and asylum in the UK* (Centre for Policy Studies, 2001) and *No System to Abuse: immigration and health care in the UK* (CPS 2003). She has also written three books: *Between the Lines: Conversations in South Africa* describes the effect of apartheid on some of its Indian, coloured, black and Afrikaaner inhabitants in the early 1980s. *Shanghai* is a history of the world's most international city between 1927 and 1939. *The Old Sow in the Back Room* recounts her experiences of Tokyo where she stayed for seven years. She has written for numerous newspapers and magazines in Britain and abroad.

*Support towards research for this Study
was given by the Institute for Policy Research.*

ISBN No. 1 903219 65 5

CONTENTS

Preface

1. Introduction   1

2. The Chief Executive   14

3. Middle Management   37

4. Front-line Managers   63

5. Infection in the NHS hospital   85

6. Conclusions   92

PREFACE

THIS REPORT takes a fresh look at management in the National Health Service. It is based on extensive interviews and research over an eleven month period. I was fortunate to have the co-operation of six very different hospitals. Three are in London, one on London's outer circle, one in a university town and a rural hospital in the West Country. I interviewed chairmen, chief executives, middle management, consultants, matrons, sisters, nurses, porters, cleaners and, of course, patients. I sat in on management meetings and shadowed front-line staff. I also did volunteer work in my local hospital and have arrived as a patient at Accident and Emergency departments more than half a dozen times.

The surprising factor was the level of agreement in these very different hospitals.

Over and over again people complained of the same thing often at odds with government and top management pronouncements. I would be told of impressive, new initiatives. Then I would go onto the wards and hear from patients a very different story; of long waits, bad food and dirty lavatories.

The observations I make are not based on a comprehensive survey. Three years ago the Department of Health itself admitted it did not even know how many managers it employed or what their roles were. This year they have changed their definition of an NHS manager to make the increase in their numbers, one suspects, less obvious.

The NHS is a very large organisation. There is enormous variety in the quality of hospitals and patient care received from one town to the next, from one doctor to the next and even from one nurse to the next. There is an equally enormous variety in the quality of NHS management. I believe the observations I make here give a fair picture of an organisation struggling to be better – but an organisation that is fundamentally flawed and in need of a new approach.

CHAPTER ONE

INTRODUCTION

YOU ARE LYING on a trolley in casualty. You have been lying there a long time. You are in pain and in shock. Your well-organised life is in chaos. You are stripped of control. You are being treated like an imbecile and are called by your Christian name. You cannot use your mobile phone or reach the outside world. You have just discovered the indignity of a bedpan. For the first time since you were a baby, you are powerless and dependent.

Unlike infancy, no one cares or comes when you call. Everyone is busy with something else. Young doctors stare at computer screens. Nurses hurry past or reply brusquely. The place is shabby and chaotic. No one appears to be in control or have authority. You have entered a time warp and been transported back to an era where consumer choice and individual rights count for nothing. Automatically you adjust your outlook to that of a supplicant. A tramp, his blackened feet on display, has started to sing. In a corner a young man is banging his head against the wall.

You may have been mugged, had a car accident or a heart attack. Whatever the cause, you are the latest victim of the NHS and, in particular, the problem of managing an NHS hospital. It is not for want of numbers. Unlike doctors, nurses or radiologists, management numbers have shot up. Between 1995 and 2001, the number of senior managers has jumped by 48%, and the number of managers by 24%.

The appointment of managers has taken precedence over front-line staff. Over the same period, for example, the number of qualified nurses, has risen by a mere 7.8%.[1] Figures for the year to September 2002 shows this trend continuing. The number of managers rose by 17.5% but nurses by only 5% and doctors by 5.2%.

How many managers exist in the NHS depends on who is doing the counting and how they define a manager. Like many areas of the NHS, data is unreliable or subject to political manipulation. By one estimate there are now 270,000 managers, administrators and support people working in the NHS – rather more than one to every one of the 185,000 NHS beds.[2] Gill Morgan, chief executive of the NHS Confederation representing health service management, puts the figure at 32,000 senior managers with 90,000 staff in jobs that are 'partly managerial'. But that is only a 'best estimate'.[3]

The NHS Confederation certainly believes there is a problem. In an effort to launch a debate on 'Rethinking Performance Management' in the NHS, its *Leading Edge* briefings states:[4]

> The current system appears to fail both the performance managers and those they manage; neither does it directly connect to front-line clinicians or their patients.

So too does the Secretary of State for Health. He said:[5]

> The problem lies not with doctors, nurses, cleaners or other staff, but the management and organisation of the hospitals.

Indifferent, poorly trained nurses, unmotivated auxiliary nurses, absent porters, dirty wards, embittered consultants, lost patient notes, hospital acquired infections, broken or lost equipment, disorganised discharge, waste and inferior treatment are all indicative of bad management, or, no management at all.

---

[1]   The full figures can be found at the Department of Health website: www.doh.gov.uk/public/nhsworkforce/sb0202.xls.

[2]   For numbers of NHS beds see: www.doh.gov.uk/hpsss/tbl_B16.htm

[3]   Quoted in *The Guardian*, 25 June 2003.

[4]   NHS Confederation, *Leading Edge 2*, page 1, 2001.

[5]   Quoted in the NHS Confederation evidence to Select Committee on Public Administration on targets.

INTRODUCTION

The Government is betting that more money will deliver higher standards. Certainly funding is an issue. But so is proper management. There is a huge gap between what the Government says is happening and the experience of the ordinary patient. This gap is caused by the inability of hospital management to manage.

At every level, from the chief executive through middle managers to managers on the front line, management is often either ineffectual or absent. Why this is so and its devastating affect on the patient is the remit of this paper.

This Government has staked its reputation on delivering a vastly improved NHS. In its report *Achieving the NHS Plan,* published in June this year,[6] the Audit Commission points out that the internal management capacity of NHS trusts, 'will be fundamental' to how they will 'respond to the Plan's future challenges.' So what is going wrong with NHS management?

"I don't think I have ever seen a manager"

It is a revelation to anyone spending time in a hospital to discover how little of hospital activity is actually managed. There is a perception that there is too much management and that it is too intrusive. This might be so amongst top and middle management. But when you work your way down through the strata of NHS hospital management, you make a discovery. The closer you get to the patient, the less management there is.

The people who have the most contact with the patient, front-line staff such as consultants, housemen, nurses, cleaners and porters are either, as one consultant remarked recently 'in open warfare' with management or hardly managed at all.

Initiatives 'cascade down' as managers are eager to tell you but the return journey appears more problematic. 'I don't think I have ever seen a manager,' said one young houseman as if talking of a mythical species. He had a plan for streamlining his hospital's chaotic blood sampling system but no idea who to approach.

---

6   Audit Commission, *Achieving the NHS Plan,* 2003.

Private hospitals employ far more managers at the sharp end – as one general manager of a BUPA hospital said, 'Everyone knows their managers' – but far fewer managers overall. There are, according to Dr Maurice Slevin, consultant medical oncologist at Barts, four and a half times as many managers, administrators and support staff to nurses in the NHS as in the private sector. He concludes:[7]

> If a private hospital was to have the same management-nurse ratio as the NHS it would either have to recruit a further 143 management, administrative and support staff; or sack 186 of their 240 nurses.

The problems of NHS management are exacerbated by what the NHS Confederation has called the 'disconnected hierarchy' of NHS management.[8] The NHS Confederation has stated that the top of the organisation 'is not effectively connected to the front line and may not even share the same objectives and priorities.'

The disconnection is there for all to see. In most hospitals it is a physical fact. Management nearly always work in a separate wing or building to the hospital segregated by a lawn, a tennis court or, in one case, a Japanese garden. They are tranquil, often attractive places that have little in common with the hospitals they serve.

An insuperable barrier appears to exist between them and their front-line staff. Chief executives of two and three star hospitals talked of incentives for their staff, of tea parties and diplomas. But not one member of staff that I questioned (except a porter in a zero rated star hospital on the edge of London) had ever heard of these rewards – let alone been presented with one.

Bring back matron?

This lack of management is reflected in the call heard over and over again from patients and staff alike for the return of the 'good, old

---

7   M Slevin, *Resuscitating the NHS*, Centre for Policy Studies, 2003.
8   NHS Confederation, *Leading Edge 2*, page 4, 2001.

fashioned' matron. In effect, this is a call for a return to strong leadership at patient level that is capable of taking responsibility to make and carry through decisions and that sees no boundary between the clinical and the managerial. Or, as the NHS Plan puts it 'with authority to get basics right on the ward.' Someone to get the lavatories cleaned, to see old people are eating properly, to supervise the training of junior nurses and to provide an assessment of every patient to the consultant on his ward round. Someone who has the power to give orders in numerous different spheres of hospital activity for one end only – the comfort and well-being of their patient. This is what the NHS claims to want and what the Government is putting our money into achieving.

Unfortunately no one, from the chief executive down, enjoys that boundary-leaping authority. Political correctness, the power of the unions and centrally set targets all take precedence over the well-being of patients. Their care is almost incidental in the process.

NHS management lack the basic tools of management. They cannot reward the excellent. Nor can they sack the incompetent (or not without great difficulty). Instead miscreants are promoted, re-employed in another job (chief executives tend to go to the Department of Health, nurses into out-patient care, and porters to catering) or, at the most, reprimanded 'in a soft voice' as one former matron described and 'offered a training course'.

The lack of management authority reveals itself in the sheer, arbitrary nature of NHS care. A patient will experience in one day, often in one hour, disorganisation and indifference side by side with first-class care and illuminating kindness. This is what makes criticism of the NHS so difficult. For every tale of horror is another of exceptional service. It is not the quality of care that is at issue but its randomness. There is little incentive for a nurse to check an old lady for bedsores except her own humanity and professionalism. Nor is there any punishment if she forgets or does not bother.

"Articulate and empowered patients"?

At a conference on 'Empowering Patients' in 2001 Hazel Blears MP, the then Parliamentary Under-Secretary of State for Health called for the creation of 'articulate and empowered' patients as vital 'to improve standards' and to bring about 'a cultural change' in the service. Apart from making it sound as if one must pass an exam before entering hospital, it also reveals little understanding of what it is like to fall ill. No one is articulate and empowered on a bedpan. No one is articulate or empowered when they have been told that they have six months to live, or they have to undergo even a minor operation or they are in pain. Patients are vulnerable and dependent. That is what illness does to you. That is why good management is vital.

The arbitrary nature of care in the NHS falls hardest on those people least able to stand up for themselves. The NHS has generated many myths but the myth that we all receive equal service is the most pernicious. In a poorly managed hospital, it is a free for all. The meek and the ignorant are made to wait, get overlooked and receive, as I saw, bad and often life threatening treatment. The well connected, the middle class and the obstreperous jump the queue.

This is hard to accept. Since its inception in 1949 the NHS has exerted a powerful hold on the nation. Its fairness defines us. It is a source of pride and comfort that people receive free medical treatment. Nigel Lawson has described it as 'the closest thing the English have to a religion.'

The NHS has acted as a force for social cohesion. In many cases it still does. A number of people described the friendships made in their six bed bay during their stay – often because they had to nurse and care for each other. Nick Bosanquet, Professor of Health Policy at Imperial College, University of London, talks of the 'important human commitment' the NHS represents. He goes on 'but surely such an aspiration will be devalued, even hopelessly compromised, if we are not prepared to asses the actual results that are achieved in practice.' To make a moral commitment and then not to consider alternative ways of reaching it is 'paradoxical and irresponsible.'[9]

This is exactly the position that hospital management finds itself in – a moral commitment to care for patients but not the tools to ensure that care.

"A lack of real world delivery experience"

Targets are meant to enable them to do just that. The Government is castigated for its emphasis on targets. But not all targets are bad. Indeed, the kind of targets the Government is setting are often commendable. They represent a shift in emphasis from the cost to the quality of health care.

It is not always the targets themselves that cause concern but their sheer number – and the number of new administrators needed to monitor them. The NHS Plan promised 'to root out unnecessary administrative cost' and to spend money, 'on the right things – front-line care.' At the same time it set 186 targets in just 144 pages.[10] Monitoring and evaluating requires people.

Again and again, chief executives told me their first priority was to appoint a new manager to ensure they were complying with the latest government initiative. The management board meeting I attended was almost wholly taken up with discussing compliance. The Government has created a Kafkaesque situation. Hospitals are recruiting more and more managers to monitor care which fails to improve partly because of their appointment.

It is not a new situation. Nearly every reform of the NHS has led to an increase in administrative staff. The formation of NHS management itself was the result of just such an exercise. In 1983 the Thatcher Government asked Roy Griffiths, Managing Director of Sainsbury's to look at manpower in the NHS. Each previous

---

9   N Bosanquet, *A Successful National Health Service*, ASI, 1999.

10   G Clark and J Mather, *Total Politics*, Conservative Policy Unit, 2003.

reform during the 1960s and 1970s had seen an increase in manpower. The changes introduced by Keith Joseph in 1974 had needed, for example, a 30% increase in clerical and administrative staff. By the early 1980s some local health authorities admitted they had no idea how many staff they employed.[11]

Griffiths pointed out that a problem with manpower meant a problem with management. His conclusion applies even more today, 'If Florence Nightingale was carrying her lamp through the corridors of the NHS today,' he wrote, 'she would almost certainly be searching for the people in charge.'

He urged that managers should replace administrators. A line-management system was created, running from civil servants in the Department of Health all the way down to what was to become the ward manager. This new system was intended to provide politicians with a lever which, when manipulated by the centre, produced results on the ward. Without Griffiths, the later reforms could not have happened. There would have been no one to deliver them. They also provided ministers and civil servants with an unprecedented chance to interfere. This political interference has had a calamitous effect on hospital management.

Central direction is inspired by the best of intentions. Whitehall very properly wants to improve standards. In the market place this is done by the customer dithering over different brands of dog food. Unfortunately the NHS user is denied that choice. Whitehall's problem is how to replicate the effects of customer choice. Civil servants appear to believe that challenging targets results in change. The NHS Plan offers an elaborate quality-improvement process driven by inspectors. But too many targets see the system falter. There are only so many on which an organisation can concentrate. When resources are limited there have to be trade-offs. Whitehall appears not to have understood this.

---

[11]   N Timmins, *The Five Giants: A Biography of the Welfare State*, HarperCollins, 1995.

INTRODUCTION

James Strachan, Chairman of the Audit Commission remarked in his evidence to the Select Committee on Public Administration of targets, 'There is a dire need to train people in how to set these targets, and to train people in how to use them.' The people setting targets at the senior level suffer from, 'a lack of real world delivery experience and this is shown time and time again.'

Is it possible to start and sustain the changes demanded by the NHS Plan without the discipline of the market place? Alain Enthoven, Professor of Public and Private Management at Stanford University and the intellectual architect of previous Conservative reforms, points to business people who have turned around failing companies speaking of 'near-death experiences' as they realised their competitors were about to destroy them. He adds that it is much harder to reform a public sector monopoly because there is no competition, no 'near-death experience to get people's attention and make them want to change.'[12]

The NHS is above all a vast bureaucracy. Like any bureaucracy, the NHS has a history of hijacking policies that are supposed to benefit the patient, to its own purposes. The NHS Plan has this in common with every other attempt to reform the NHS over the last 54 years. All the good intentions will come to one end – to expand and strengthen what Alan Milburn called in its introduction, 'a culture where the convenience of the patient can come a poor second to the convenience of the system.'

"I felt I had got lost in a maze with no chance of escaping"
The Government calls again and again for 'a patient-centred service'. But how many people who make decisions on our healthcare have actually been a patient of the NHS? How many people working in the NHS itself have been a patient?

Labour Ministers make a point of using the NHS but their experience is hardly typical. The wife of a member of the Cabinet,

---

[12]   *British Journal of Health Care Management*, Vol 7 No. 2, 2001.

for example, had a minor operation on the NHS. She by-passed the waiting list and, for security reasons, did not go on the ward but had her own room. When she left, she presented her nurses with a bottle of bubble bath, 'As if she thought we all took our baths together,' remarked one.

Civil Servants at the Ministry of Health are entitled, for example, to become a member of the Benenden Healthcare Society which serves one million British Telecom, Post Office and Civil Service workers and their families. They can stay in its privately-run hospital in the Kent countryside, and as different as you can get from an NHS hospital.

At a conference on waiting lists attended by 100 NHS managers, Professor Nick Bosanquet took a show of hands on the delegates' experience of waiting lists. Only one out of the 100 had even been on one.[13] Even consultants employed by the NHS are wary of using it. One who has worked in the NHS for 20 years said, 'In the past we all knew we would get good care on the NHS. Five years ago I took out private medical insurance for my family. That's what I think of the NHS.'

Trade unions passionately defend the NHS and denounce even the modest reforms by this Government. Recently the GMB ran full-page press adverts to underline the point. A smiling nurse stood next to a young executive. 'Who would you prefer to run the NHS?' read the caption. The TUC has certainly made its choice. In the past Bill Morris, leader of the TGWU, and John Monks, General Secretary of the TUC, enjoyed private medical insurance. A host of trade unions have done deals with private, independent sector organisations such as BUPA, Benenden Hospital, Medicash, SimplyHealth and Standard Life. They acknowledge the shortcomings of the NHS by offering membership of a private healthcare scheme as a perk to members.

---

13   N Bosanquet, op. cit.

INTRODUCTION

More than 3.5 million of the TUC's 6.8 million members now hold some form of private medical insurance. It is a higher proportion than any other socio-economic group in the UK. Unison, the biggest trade union in Britain representing people who work in public services, displays on its web site what it wishes to deny to the general public: membership of a private health benefit scheme. Unison members like NHS porters, for example, can join Medicash which offers cash to those who need medical care. The Essential Surgery Plan, which, we are reassured on its website, is 'Unison approved', protects against the cost and inconvenience of undergoing surgery 'either on the NHS or privately'. Members can receive £400 to £6,000 a year for an operation, 'giving you the freedom to choose how, when or where you're treated – or spend the money how you wish if your treatment is undertaken by the NHS!'

A surprising number of people who work in healthcare have no experience of being a patient. One consultant who had obviously never been ill himself described in amazement the transformation in his patients, 'What I thought was innate to their character, depression, irritability, lack of confidence, was actually due to their illness.'

A woman seconded to the Department of Health was astonished to find few of her colleagues had actually worked in a hospital, let alone been a patient. A manager in charge of the complaints system in a London hospital found being ill in his own hospital illuminating. 'I had no idea what it was like to be a patient even though I work with them. I know the system but even I got into difficulties finding out who my doctor was, what medicine to take and when I was getting out. I lay there helpless. I felt I had got lost in a maze with no chance of escaping.'

IT DOES NOT HAVE TO BE LIKE THIS

BENENDEN HOSPITAL: A CASE STUDY

After spending eleven months visiting NHS hospitals, Benenden Hospital, surrounded by the Kent countryside with its tennis court, swimming pool and farm, its large, airy rooms and balconies with views over lawns studded with cedar trees is like stepping into paradise. Around each nurse station, the walls are smothered with cards from grateful patients many embroidered and framed. 'You made me feel very special' and 'I would have liked to stay longer,' read the messages of praise and gratitude.

This paradise is not for the general public Benenden healthcare is for employees and their families of The Post Office, Civil Service, BT, the education sector, local authorities and other approved public bodies who are under 64 and a half at the time of enrolment. It has over a million members. It provides consultations, medical and surgical treatment and cancer care support at its own hospital in Kent and through a network of independent hospitals throughout the UK. No medical is required to join. There are no exclusions for pre-existing conditions and no increase in contributions with age. Everyone pays the same rate per person per week of an extraordinarily cheap 95p. As one member pointed out, she pays in a year for The Benenden Healthcare what private medical insurance costs her brother in one month.

It is clear why Benenden Healthcare works. It is not a front-line provider of healthcare nor private insurance. It is a genuine mutual benefit organisation. As it states in its Members News letter 'Our service is not based on claiming on anything that you can; it is based on trust and mutual aid. It is your society and we trust that you will use it responsibly.'

Benenden's funds are provided on a discretionary basis. By law it is not compelled to provide anything to anyone. In fact there is a very low take up by members Bill McPate, its Projects Director explained, 'This would not work for the general public. Our members are responsible. They feel if they are not benefiting, they are still happy to pay because someone else is. This kind of Mutual Society only works for a group with a strong sense of responsibility.'

One man recounted his experience. He was told an operation was out of the question because he did not have enough oxygen in the blood. 'At that point I thought of committing suicide.' He remembered he was a member of Benenden Healthcare and approached them. He was offered treatment at Benenden hospital. His daughter drove him down from Grimsby to Kent by car 'we were that desperate'. During the second week he seized Bill Pate by the hand, 'Feel that,' he said. 'So?' Bill Pate said. The old man replied, 'My hands are warm – the first time in 20 years.' Shortly after he was well enough to have the operation.

One woman with a stomach complaint pointed out that on the NHS she would have had to wait months between every test, 'It would have taken 18 months. Here I have had all my tests done in two weeks.'

Benenden is not trying to replace the NHS. It is instead offering choice. When I asked a retired postman on a ward in Benenden what he thought of his private hospital, he replied firmly, 'it's not a private hospital, it's a worker's hospital, our hospital' He defines public ownership as ownership by Benenden's members – not an administrative class in Whitehall.

It is a great pity that trade unions are not promoting more Benendens.

CHAPTER TWO

THE CHIEF EXECUTIVE

IN THE PORTERS' ROOM of a One Star hospital on the edge of London, flanked by posters of half-naked girls, hung this notice:

> ATTENTION! Running a company is simple. I should know.
> I'm running yours.

The lack of managerial authority starts at the top. The chief executive of an NHS Trust or hospital enjoys a unique position. He is the only person in his hospital whose position is precarious. Consultants, for example, have a job effectively for life. Getting rid of them, as one Human Resource Manager put it is, 'a huge, great whacking procedure' Incapable nurses (either through sickness, injury or just incompetence) are offered alternative work. 'We have to exhaust every option to provide them with another career,' explained the Human Resource Manager. Cleaners and porters are protected by their powerful union, Unison.

The chief executive, on the other hand has a far less secure status. He is at the whim of Whitehall, a victim of an NHS subject to political intervention and easy to sacrifice if some problem affecting the trust attracts bad publicity. Turnover is high. In 2001 nearly one in five NHS chief executives left or were replaced. The rate I encountered was even higher. Of the four chief executives that I interviewed, three have since left their hospitals. Hoggett Bowers, the executive search consultancy, notes the typical tenure of an NHS chief executive is 700 days.[14] 'The life of the chief executive,' as

---

[14]   Hoggett Bowers website.

one with experience in the public sector put it, 'is nasty, brutish and short.'[15] Or, as Hoggett Bowers says, a 'white-knuckle ride.'

This hardly encourages the strong and effective leadership required to run a hospital and to safeguard patients' interests. One chief executive of a leading London hospital explained how it affected her (and, ironically, the only one I interviewed still in her post):

> The average life span in this job is two and a half years. So I can't afford to concentrate on just my hospital. I have to get myself another portfolio. I have to spend a good deal of my time out there networking.

At the same time the chief executive of an NHS hospital carries a heavy burden. The Health Act of 1999 made it the duty of each health authority, trust and primary care trust to put and keep in place arrangements for the purpose of monitoring and improving the quality of the health care it provides. For the first time, trusts and their chief executives were responsible and accountable for the quality of care in their hospitals. In order to discharge this responsibility, 'they must', as the Bristol Royal Infirmary Inquiry Report pointed out, 'be given the tools for the job.'[16] Instead they find themselves caught in a vice. At the same time as Whitehall exerts a capricious and demanding authority over them, they are unable to exert the same authority over their own staff.

"A string of arrogant messages from the centre"

Chief executives, whether of successful Three Star hospitals or hospitals with no stars at all, whether of inner city or a rural hospital in the West country, all made the same complaint. They suffered from Whitehall's 'overbearing presence' and its demand

---

[15]   Quoted in the *Report of the Public Inquiry into children's heart surgery at the Bristol Royal Infirmary 1985-1994* (hereafter the Bristol Public Inquiry Report), July 2001.

[16]   Ibid., Chapter 24.

for information, form-filling and target-setting estimated, according to the NHS Confederation 'at over 400 for a Primary Care Trust and over 250 for an acute trust'.[17]

One chief executive of a One Star hospital in a university town described how five years before he had spent 5% of his time on 'upward management'. Now, responding to 'a string of arrogant messages from the centre' took up 20% of his time. He gave an example. That day the Ministry of Health had e-mailed him wanting five points on waiting list times answered by 11 a.m. the following morning. As chief executive, it was his job to demand that information from his operational manager. 'It's micro-management to a ridiculous level.'

The chief executive of a Three Star hospital in the West country made the same complaint. The week after Milburn made his speech on foundation hospitals, they received a letter from Whitehall. Were they interested in foundation status? The note arrived on Tuesday. They had to prepare a response by 5 p.m. on Wednesday. The chief executive dismissed this as far too short a time. 'A fundamental decision like this needs serious thought. I would want to discuss it with my board.' Whitehall often required a response in just three hours. As the chief executive remarked, 'You don't have time to think through decisions. You are just fire-fighting.' The finance director of a Zero Star hospital on the edge of London complained that Whitehall's demands for 'a detailed plan of action' meant that time better spent on thought was wasted conjuring up a time table, 'which you have no idea if you can keep to.'

Another chief executive pointed out that four or five years ago, his hospital had to achieve fewer than 20 targets, 'and we were pretty clear what the big ones were.' Since then performance targets have risen to 'a ridiculous level.' At any one time he is responsible for achieving 420 targets. He tried to write them down

---

[17]   Memorandum (PST 13) to the Select Committee on Public Administration submitted by the NHS Confederation.

on one piece of paper – 'but we could not get them all on.' Another pointed out that, amongst the 40 human resources targets that he has to meet, he must give the percentage of his staff who have received an appraisal for their personal development plan. 'That is part of my job. If I don't do it then I am a bad manager. But why insult me by checking? If the Department of Health doesn't trust me, why did they give me the job in the first place?' Another wanted Whitehall to pick two or three key measures that, 'I can hold in my head and my managers can hold in their heads. And come down hard on those.'

Sir Nigel Crisp, chief executive of the NHS, admitted in January 2003 to the Select Committee on Public Administration that the volume of targets had become burdensome. He proposed reducing the number of targets from April this year to 62 with 26 further 'assumptions about capacity' – not quite the five or six that the NHS Confederation thinks is the maximum and 'the key to the whole system.'[18]

Sir Nigel Crisp is also responsible for the Leadership Centre of the NHS Modernisation Agency, established with a budget of £150 million a year. Its latest portfolio, the result of almost 12 months of work reviewing and reviving previous initiatives, offers 'challenging, stimulating and effective opportunities' for chief executives to learn new skills. The Modernisation Agency is clear what these should be – and they are not to do with running a hospital.

The NHS is above all an organisation subject to political pressure. Out of the nine 'skills development,' courses offered, the top five concentrate on the chief executive's relationship with government, Whitehall and the media. So a chief executive can learn about 'Policy Making and How to influence it', 'The Select Committee Process,' and the 'Westminster Experience' which includes 'How Ministers operate' and, the no doubt invaluable for

---

[18]   NHS Confederation, *Leading Edge 3*, 2001.

the much put-upon NHS chief executive, 'How to use a crises involving Ministers/Whitehall positively.'

As one chief executive said sadly, 'More and more I realise what my job is really about is politics. We are an extension of the civil service.'

"The carrots are so small that you can't make them into things that people would consume for nourishment"

The chief executive might be at the beck and call of Whitehall. He is, however, unable to exert the same authority over his staff. In a company every employee is a member who can be rewarded or fired. In a hospital the loyalty of the various organised occupations and professions may lie as much outside, to a Royal College for example, as to the hospital itself. The NHS contains powerful professional groups, particularly medicine, with a long history of influence and independence whose primary allegiance is to individual patients rather than collective or corporate objectives set by management. Chief executives who stay a few years can hardly command the same loyalty from consultants and nurses whose appointments are stable and long-term.

In a series of seminars organised by The Bristol Royal Infirmary Inquiry, the various participants who came from organisations other than the NHS were surprised by the complexity of employment relationships in the NHS. They noted that 'a chief executive and a trust's board can be disempowered by strong professional groupings, apparently beyond the chief executive's control to manage. They also observed that doctors 'do not respond to senior management' but to professional peers whom they respect and 'who may not even be in the same organisation.'[19]

Sir Stanley Kalms, the former chairman of Dixons and one of the country's most successful entrepreneurs, was chairman of an NHS hospital in London. He found himself up against 'a large, self-protected bureaucracy' and a medical staff 'as powerful as

---

[19]   *The Bristol Royal Infirmary Inquiry Report.*

medieval barons'. He went on, 'It is not an easy job unless the chief executive is all powerful'. But that is the problem. The chief executive of one North London hospital who has worked in the private sector had expected to find 'the pulls and levers you have in industry'. Instead the NHS provides, 'a much more informal structure' of command. 'Informal' is the best he can hope for when he lacks the essential tools of management to, as Sir Stanley Kalms remarked, 'hire, fire and kick butts.'

Even something as minor as holidays remains out of the chief executive's control. At the management board meeting of one north London hospital the chief executive declared himself 'slightly astonished' to discover the hospital did not 'honestly know' how much leave consultants were taking or when they were taking it. There was no attempt to stagger leave. At certain times so many doctors were away without a replacement, it affected waiting lists. 'It's all got very confused,' said the chief executive, 'we need a few bullet points.'

Motivation of staff is another problem for the chief executive of an NHS hospital. His own is far from transparent. Information on the earnings of NHS chief executives lags far behind the standards of disclosure in the private sector. In the financial year ending in March, 2002, remuneration for chief executives varied according to trust size from £72,500 to £114,500. More than half of NHS trust chief executives could have received double figure percentage salary rises last year and nearly a quarter 20% or more. But no one outside the hospital boardrooms will ever know. As a result of a change of policy, NHS trusts are no longer obliged to give out precise figures. A rise in salaries has seen a decline in bonus payments. Only a handful of chief executives received bonuses. How and why NHS chief executives get a salary raise or a bonus is in many cases a 'closed book' according to Incomes Data Services. Sometimes it is just the result of a surplus in trust income.[20]

---

[20]   Incomes Data Services, *The NHS Boardroom Pay Report*, 2003.

Chief executives might receive raises but they are not allowed to award them to their staff. Consultants receive merit awards but this is opaquely determined by other consultants. As Sir Stanley Kalms remarked, 'The carrots are so small that you can't make them into things that people would consume for nourishment.' An anaesthetist consultant at a London teaching hospital recalled his last annual encounter with his department. He described the 100 procedures he had completed, all of them successfully. He did not receive a word of praise, let alone a bonus. How would the successful executive of a private company react to similar treatment? NHS chief executives have to fall back on the occasional tea party or diploma.

"So and So is incompetent," "Yes but they are awfully nice"
The ability to fire people is another essential management tool. But this too is denied the NHS chief executive – or at least made very difficult. The NHS does not encourage confrontation and nastiness. As one chief executive put it, 'We are a caring profession. But sometimes we put caring for our colleagues above caring for our patients.'

Sir Stanley Kalms said, 'The system does not eject. It is a great evil in the system,' He decided to give a series of tea parties for long serving staff. The party to celebrate those who had worked in the hospital for 25 years proved a revelation. Neither he nor anyone else in the hospital had ever seen the majority who turned up. Some were ill, others grotesquely overweight, all 'no longer fit and proper people to be in a hospital.' But they were all still on the pay roll.

They were sisters, nurses or auxiliary nurses. Further up the hierarchy, it is hardly any different. A senior non-executive director described some of the managers in her trust as, 'not up to the job.' This did not mean she could sack them. 'The NHS,' she explained, 'does not like facing noise.' Another remarked, 'Time and time again I have said, "So and So is incompetent," only to be reproved, "Yes but they are awfully nice."' The easiest way of getting rid of these 'awfully nice' people in an organisation as huge as the NHS is to promote them somewhere else. Special project work 'paper clip projects,' as one Human Resource Manager described it, or, 'refiguring the system' proved popular. 'Amazing how much crap gets put forward for that,' remarked the senior non-executive director. She was in London for a meeting when she discovered a 'dire chap' she had wanted to sack in the next door office. He had just started inspecting for Commission for Health Improvement (CHI).

Promoting an inept colleague is always at the expense of the patient. In December 2001, the National Audit Commission published a report on nine NHS trusts which had fiddled their waiting lists.[21] This affected 6,000 patient records. In serious cases patients were 'inappropriately suspended,' never put on or just removed from waiting lists. 'If action had not been taken,' stated the Audit Office, 'the trusts had no mechanisms in place to ensure that all these patients received the treatment they needed.' In other words patients were left, for years in some cases, in pain, their condition deteriorating, still believing that they were on a waiting list.

What happened to the senior managers and chief executives concerned? 'Most of the individuals,' states the report, 'have found re-employment within the NHS.' In five of the nine trusts those found guilty received generous payments (in two cases £146,000) then, incredibly, went on to find new jobs within the NHS. In the majority of cases their references, as the National Audit Office put it, 'made no mention of inappropriate adjustment,' to waiting lists and even contained a confidentiality clause 'inconsistent,' as the report pointed out, 'with the proper conduct of public business.' Some of the new NHS employers were 'aware of circumstances.' It did not seem a drawback. This reluctance to punish and expel transgressors does neither staff moral or patients any favours.

---

[21]   National Audit Office, *Inappropriate Adjustments to NHS Waiting Lists*, 2001.

"A very distracting add-on irritant"

The chief executive of a hospital spends a great deal of time gathering information for Whitehall's 400 or so targets. But how much of that information does what it should do? Which is to help the chief executive run his hospital. Many chief executives found they hit the targets but failed their patients and their hospitals.

Targets divert the chief executive's attention from what is happening in his own hospital. In his evidence to the Select Committee on Public Administration, James Strachan, Chairman of the Audit Commission said of targets that far from being an integrated part of day-to-day management, they can become 'a very distracting add-on irritant.'

One of the chief executive's most important targets is the number of cancer patients who are seen within two weeks of visiting their GP. This appears to be a good target. It is clear and simple to measure from the point the patient sees the GP to the point they are seen in hospital. However it distorts the picture both for the chief executive and for the patient. It misses what is vital to the patient which is not when he sees the consultant, but when he starts his treatment. It causes delays further up the system because the hospital has concentrated on the target. The patient sees the consultant, learns he has cancer and then has to wait an indeterminate amount of time for radiotherapy or chemotherapy for which there is no target, 'like re-arranging the decks on the Titanic,' as one radiologist said when asked to fit in another patient. A more appropriate target would be to measure the time it takes from that first appointment with the GP to finishing treatment. That would allow the chief executive and his cancer team to rethink the whole process and not just a bit of it.

An inspector for the Audit Commission pointed out that information gathered is for government consumption – not to enable chief executives to make a decision. 'They are gathering the wrong sort of information and, in my experience, not using it effectively. There is a lack of vision and strategy.' In its submission to the Public Administration Select Committee, the NHS Confederation stated that 'there is a real problem that the civil service conception of managerially useful information does not reflect the realities of how organisations are actually run'. Or as one consultant put it, 'Why are we being told what to do by 30 year olds with no experience of life who have obviously never set foot in a hospital?' The non-executive director of one NHS Trust dismissed most information-gathering by his NHS chief executive as, 'a smoke screen'. He went on, 'if a piece of information does not lead to a decision, then it's not worth collecting.'

The blizzard of information can blind the chief executive to what is good for his patients. Targets themselves cannot produce useful management information. Information systems need to be in place to produce reliable data. The inspector for the Audit Commission noted that a number of chief executives of hospitals that he visited knew the cost of a treatment but not the value. They remained unaware of the clinical outcome – how the operation has benefited the patient over the long term. The Audit Commission itself noted that too often targets are 'focused on the stages and processes' of delivering health care rather than 'on the outcome for the patient.'[22] As the Bristol Royal Infirmary Inquiry discovered, 'There is very little, good quality, outcome data for clinical procedures'.[23] Its collection receives little support or resources in the NHS. What data does exist is not easily translated into usable information.

This information is vital to the patient. The Audit inspector gave the example of two surgeons in a hospital he visited, both performing hip replacements. The first surgeon performed his operations faster. He could operate on more patients in a session and his waiting list was consequently shorter. Management, however, failed to measure the clinical outcome between the two

---

[22]   Submission from Audit Commission to the Select Committee on Public Administration.

[23]   *The Bristol Royal Infirmary Inquiry Report*, Summary.

men. The patients of the first surgeon needed a new hip replacement on average every five years, of the second surgeon, only every ten years. This crucial information was unavailable to the chief executive. So the first surgeon received the majority of patients – even though it would cost the hospital far more in the long run not to mention the distress of a further operation to the patient.

Why did this information remain unavailable to the chief executive? The auditor dismissed attempts to collect it as 'not robust'. The consultants – 'a closed shop of clinicians looking after themselves' – refused to provide information detrimental to a colleague. Management, unaware of its importance and overwhelmed by Department of Health's demands for other data, made no attempt to get it. Without such crucial information, feared the auditor, how could a chief executive know where lay the key issues or make progress in resolving them?

Information is a lot more than IT ware. Information is motivating people to report accurately and completely. The Audit Commission have pointed to 'the poor quality' of much of the data collected.[24] While Francis Blunden, principal policy adviser on Health for the Consumer's Association criticised the Department of Health of, 'complacency' and for failing to asses the 'quality of the data' they receive. Dr Gill Morgan, chief executive of the NHS Confederation explained, 'if you are collecting information you personally are going to use, information gets to be good. If you are collecting information to go into a black box somewhere else which you never actually, as the person collecting it, see any benefit for, we know that information becomes inaccurate.' The Department of Health is not interested in the accuracy of the information. They want figures that will satisfy the Health Minister. Figures that allow him to stand up in Parliament and answer questions with confidence – not help chief executives do their job.

---

[24]   Submission from Audit Commission to the Select Committee on Public Administration.

"A vast bureaucratic fudge of funding"

The way from money comes from government is rarely straightforward. As Sir Stanley Kalms said, 'The top-slicing of money through Whitehall is just wicked.' A certain amount of money is held back each financial year and earmarked for different areas of hospital improvement. When the Government desires some good publicity, money is suddenly available but only for certain trusts. Hospitals have to bid for these funds. One chief executive said gloomily, 'We live in a bidding culture.' These dollops of money are vital for the hospital. Another chief executive explained that his hospital received £24 million from the Government. On top of that he could bid for an extra 1% or a quarter of a million pounds. It sounds little but, 'managing in the NHS is about managing at the margin.' He explained, 'So much is fixed or semi fixed that I spend 80% of my time managing 3% or 4% of my income.' This extra cash is vital for the chief executive. As one said, 'we are going to miss targets unless we get the money.'

The procedure works like this. A hospital hears that money is available to do up reception areas. To qualify the hospital has to submit a comprehensive document within 10 days, 'far too short notice,' which requires a manager to spend two or three days work away from his normal job. One chief executive I interviewed was agonising over £153,000 promised by Whitehall in November to help with the recruitment of nurses over the winter. 'It's taken several manager days to get this and all for only £153,000!' he wailed. Nor were his troubles over. It was 18 January and he still had not received the money ten weeks before the end of the quarter. How could he use the money sensibly in such a short period? And how was he to fill in the monitoring sheet which would arrive in April, demanding an explanation of the expenditure. He said bitterly, 'If I ran my hospital the way they run me, there would be no hospital.'

The arbitrariness of the announcement means that 'any sensible finance director' has a portfolio of bids always to hand.

He then tops and tails them to suit the occasion. Even that may not be enough. Chief executives complained that Whitehall's decision making was often poor and unpredictable. This forced NHS chief executives to spend time on networking in their region to discover how much money might be available, when and for what. 'I have worked hard on my contacts,' said one finance director of a Zero Star rated hospital on the outskirts of London. He went on, 'I have to understand the way the policy winds are blowing and come up with ways of dealing with that.' This was time and energy away from his hospital.

Another chief executive of a Three Star hospital found these spasmodic gifts from the Government which arrived half way through the financial cycle 'very unhelpful'. Sometimes funds had already been allocated so the Government's sudden largesse, 'was a waste of money.' If you have just done up your reception area, you really don't need to do it again. Government demands for new procedures or equipment proved equally unhelpful. The Government provided one hospital with £750,000 for an MIR scanner. But as the chief executive pointed out, 'it cost us £1.1 million to install. Running costs are on top of that. The extra has to come out of our capital programme. So we have to cut out something else.' Her hospital found itself continually prioritising spending. They did not know when money was coming down, how it was coming down or what would be ring-fenced. Or what extra things Whitehall might demand they do. The Government had issued guidelines that theatre gowns used in operations should be thrown away afterwards. 'They don't say we have to do it. We did a risk assessment and decided it was a good idea for the control of infection. We made the decision but received no money for it.'

The arrival of each new initiative sees the chief executive puzzle over which to prioritise. Last week's, last month's and last year's are all sold by Whitehall as vitally important at the time. 'The trick,' as one chief executive admitted, 'is knowing when an initiative – on which we have spent money and time – has fallen out of fashion in Whitehall and can be quietly forgotten.'

Even the Department of Health admits some targets are more important than others. The NHS Confederation in its evidence to the Public Administration Select Committee explains that the Department of Health, 'encourages competitive behaviour between programmes which includes target setting'. This can lead, 'in some cases' to 'informal briefing by one part of the Department of Health against others about which are the 'real' targets and which can be ignored. This situation, described by the Chairman of the Select Committee as 'astonishing', arises because no systematic process exists from 'bottom up' to calculate how much it costs to achieve a target. Resources and targets are not matched together.

The chief executive cannot afford to implement all the various targets. So, in the peculiar NHS world where, as Frank Dobson remarked, 'everything is a priority and nothing is a priority', the chief executive of an NHS hospital asks himself one important question 'I can't afford to fulfil all these targets. So which five targets can I be sacked for?' The five, to do with access and waiting times, therefore immediately take priority. They are admirable targets. They make a difference to patients. But they mean that other things get less attention. They mean the chief executive looks at his hospital piecemeal and not as a whole.

Whitehall, quite properly, insists that hospitals meet certain financial targets. One of the criteria for Star status is financial probity. Sir Stanley Kalms looked through the figures for his hospital and called a panic meeting of the board. It was obvious they were going to fail their targets. They had to take drastic action, maybe even close a ward. His finance director, a man with long experience of working in the NHS, took a more relaxed approach, 'It will be alright on the night,' he reassured his Chairman. And it was.

Between the hospital, the trust and the then local health authority, it is important that the hospital performs. 'No one wants a hospital on their patch that does not perform,' remarked Sir Stanley Kalms, 'It really was a big game that you went through.' A finance director whose hospital did fail, put it down to the poor relationship his new chief executive had with their local health authority. 'It was purely a political decision. Our finances were in no worse state than any other London hospital'. Sir Stanley dismissed the whole thing, 'as a vast bureaucratic fudge of funding.'

The emphasis on meeting targets and bidding for money hides a serious defect in the NHS hospital: the lack of financial management. The Wanless Report states that taxpayers money must be used efficiently and effectively and recommends an independent audit to ensure that this is done.[25] There is, however, very little on how such good financial discipline might be achieved internally. Last year one NHS Trust overspent its equipment budget by two and a half times. This year it will be the same. Its non-executive director, who has had a career in trouble-shooting ailing companies, declared that he could easily save £200,000 just by good financial accounting. 'I told them, "I know what is needed. This is my background." It was as if I was speaking Ancient Greek.'

He was the only non-executive to have worked in the private sector. His finance director 'a nice man' who had spent his life in the NHS, saw money as a fixed element rather than a manager's tool. 'He does not say "What if?" only "What is". The non-executive found his ideas dismissed as too complicated and not applicable to a demand service funded by the government. Worse, his chief executive feared any investigation might expose failings that would leave him vulnerable to political interference. 'They put up a façade composed of ignorance and fear.' Dr Kailash Chard pointed out:

> No other organisation worth more than £45 billion would allow £100 million units (the average cost of running a hospital

───────────────────────────

25   D Wanless, *Securing our future health: taking a long-term view*, HM Treasury, 2002.

trust) to be managed by people who have little or no management background except a diploma in health management.[26]

Despite opposition, the non-executive director approached the equipment budget as he would in an ailing business. He started from basics, costing and budgeting everything from the bottom up. He was startled to discover that this had never been done in his trust. The cascade of money from the top had left people indifferent to the routine of accounting. Did the trust know what it owned? Was there an inventory? It appeared not. The trust even lacked a definition of what exactly is a piece of medical equipment. In the end he wrote out his own definition.

When someone placed a request for a wheelchair, he found it was not centrally administered. There was no effort to check if another hospital in the trust had a surplus of wheelchairs. Nor was there any effort to discover how much equipment had simply disappeared. Had patients who had been lent a Zimmer frame returned it? No one knew. No records appeared to have been kept. His own wife had received a crutch after breaking her foot. It was lying about at home unclaimed and presumably forgotten by the authorities.

This financial vagueness appeared in every area he examined. In his trust, 2,400 employers used several hundred vehicles on trust business but he was amazed to discover the trust lacked a policy on cars. Some leased cars, some owned cars and people were paid different rates per mile. There was no system or control on what vehicles the trust owned or what they spent on transport. The local energy company offered to do a free audit on their heating system. They discovered that £32,000 could be saved by merely adjusting the boiler control. But nothing had happened. The trust had no central administration for building repairs. The estates manager did

---

26   Quoted by G Day, *Management, Mutuality and Risk: Better Ways to Run the National Health Service*, Institute of Directors, 2000.

not sit on the hospital board. The non-executive said, 'The NHS does not need vast injections of money. It just needs someone on the inside to say how can we save money.'

He pointed to conferences. NHS staff at every level attend conferences and seminars. These are arranged by private companies who do good business explaining the implications of the government's latest initiative. Attitudes to conferences varied. Most staff resented a whole day away from work. Others saw it as a perk. One manager of an A&E department explained she sent her nurses on a seminar when they looked 'a bit mouldy.' Conferences do not come cheap. The one I attended cost £350. Chief executives and finance directors receive a sheaf of such invitations every month, 'all vital'. The non-executive pointed out that, with travelling and a night away, this cost the trust £1000 a head. 'I know myself that the chairman and the chief executive went to Harrogate last month and that alone cost £4000.' The non-executive suggested they save money by not attending any conferences the following year. How much money would they save? It could not be calculated because no one, he discovered, had any idea how much they spent on conferences.

'There is no reason,' he said, 'for the NHS not to be as properly managed as any other business.' The arrival of flu every winter, for example, put his hospital in a panic. Patients suffered from staff and bed shortages. But a glance at the figures showed this almost to be an annual event. Good business practice is to budget and plan for the unexpected. He went on, 'In my trust, management are constantly bewildered by the ordinary', the first sign of 'galloping stupidity'.

The finance director of a zero rated hospital on the edge of London saw it rather differently. He would have liked to budget and plan but events conspired against him. Much of his time was spent responding to the, 'hell of a lot of indicators' that come down from the centre. At that moment he was having to absorb the implications, 'of a whole new agenda about the way funds flow around the system,' which had required a day at the ubiquitous conference the week before. The financial information that he had to work with was 'less robust than I would like. The information is defective but I learn to live with it.' Every month he had to make judgements in which his assessment of the risks 'is as much artistic as mathematical.'

A high turnover of hospital staff meant he had to 'faff about identifying budget defects lower down the organisation' and spend the majority of his time 'fire fighting'. He was ten minutes late for our interview because he had 'suddenly' noticed that the deficit had shot up that month. 'We don't know why. We don't know if this is a one-off or a trend. The financial position in this hospital is so unstable that if you don't keep an eye on it, it turns around and bites you in the bum.' As he showed me out, he said miserably, 'At this stage in my career, I should be spending time on thinking up intellectual and creative solutions.' I did not have the heart to ask if he had ever sat down and defined a piece of medical equipment.

Government policy stresses the need for radical redesign, risk taking and social entrepreneurship. Indeed many of the more ambitious aspects of the NHS Plan depend on this. Unfortunately the Government's approach to performance management is often risk averse. Risk entails the possibility of failure. Failure reflects badly on the Government. So it tries to prescribe detail and minimise risk. It sets ever more targets, unable to grasp that the greater the number of piecemeal targets, the less its chief executives will take risks or come up with creative solutions.

A senior non-executive director was among many who pointed out that the bureaucracy of the NHS stifled enterprise, 'people of vision are not at liberty to implement that vision.' Another non-executive director of a Three Star hospital in the West Country described the hopes she had of her hospital. 'Then along comes a new initiative, maybe that is not part of your vision which gives you a bloody, big sweep off your chosen road.'

She, like many, foresaw capacity as her hospital's main problem, 'We have to look at our ageing population, make the right judgement and plan long-term.' But it is difficult, she explained to get money for long-term investment in the NHS. The political nature of the NHS condemns it to short-term fixes. Targets have not helped either. More than half of the trusts in England, according to the Audit Commission, have been diverting money to keep services running in the short term. They are paying private hospitals to carry out their work or making one-off payments to consultants for extra sessions. This means they are taking away money from IT and medical equipment, for example, and the future improvement of the service.

The chief executive's scope for action is also prescribed by the Government's inability to understand the difference between good and unacceptable diversity. Whitehall seems to regard all diversity as bad rather than the result of individual innovation or giving patients in that area what they want. Many chief executives felt they were just checking with compliance for official best practice rather than spotting and promoting a good idea. The Government's consultation document *Shifting the Balance of Power within the NHS* talks about the NHS being uniformly excellent and innovative without apparently noticing the contradiction. It is as if Whitehall expected one million NHS staff, standing in their shower, to be simultaneously struck by the same bright idea.[27]

How will this affect the Government's latest initiative, Foundation Hospitals? The Department of Health's own press release announcing their launch promised that, 'the best hospitals will be freed from excessive Whitehall control' – a remarkable confession of the Department's assessment of its own approach. One hopes they mean it.

Management is still a blind spot with Whitehall. The Audit Commission in its report, *Achieving the NHS Plan* points out that the

---

[27]   NHS Confederation, *Leading Edge 2*, 2001.

Government's star system for ranking hospitals fails to take into account management and financial capacity. The report judged several of the 29 trusts applying for Foundation status, 'to have weak management and financial arrangements.' Without them, warns James Strachan, the Chairman of the Audit Commission, there is a 'real risk' that 'billions of pounds' of new public money' earmarked for the Foundation trusts 'will not be maximised.'

As Val Gooding, BUPA's chief executive said at a conference on Foundation Hospitals, 'It takes an exceptionally high standard of clarity and focus to run a company without shareholders. The Government will need a high degree of political courage. If there is any fudge it will fail.'

The chief executive in a private hospital

The chief executive of a private hospital enjoys a much easier time. He is not subject to political pressure and constant intervention from the centre. The chief executives of BUPA's 35 hospitals, for example, are judged by a small number of indicators which are looked at quarterly. As one director of BUPA commented, 'We don't feel we need to second guess our hospital managers.'

Numbers also make a difference. The private hospital I visited in north London has 9,000 in-patients a year, about 80,000 to 90,000 out-patients and no Accident and Emergency department. Its NHS counterpart has 24,600 in-patients, 184,000 out-patients and a busy casualty department. Nonetheless there was much to learn from the chief executive's role and the management structure.

The first was the simplicity. The chief executive – or general manager as he is called in BUPA – had a senior management team of just three people: matron, support services manager and marketing manager. A team of ten operational managers reported to matron. In the absence of the general manager, she deputises, a sign of her importance. She is also the only other person apart from the chief executive on a bonus scheme. The fourth person reporting directly to the general manager was the chief engineer or estates manager, the man responsible for the fabric of the hospital. I heard constant complaints from NHS staff of the difficulty of getting anything fixed. In none of the NHS hospitals that I visited did an estates manager report directly to the chief executive. The general manager expressed surprise at this, 'He is a good man with a skilled team working for him. If something goes wrong on the ward, the nurse pages the estates manager and he responds immediately.'

The NHS chief executive has to pay his staff levels set nationally by the Government and agreed by the unions. In contrast the general manager had a free hand. He had to run a profitable hospital but he recognised that staff retention was crucial to that, 'I try and make remuneration so attractive that they find it difficult to go anywhere else.' He looked on the departure of a key member of staff as a personal failure.

Motivation of the general manager is clear. 'I am heavily bonused,' he explained. His bonus is potentially worth an additional 30% on top of basic salary and is dependent on him fulfilling certain key objectives. This compares to his NHS counterpart whose bonus – if there is one – is much smaller and less transparent. It raises a key question. How do you reward a chief executive in a state industry when no one has defined a successful performance? Is it compliance with government targets? Is it running a hospital according to local needs? Is it the quality of care delivered? Cost constraint? The number of patients treated? Is it meant to be all of these at once? And how to achieve success when some, if not all of the above, are mutually exclusive and the emphasis shifts every few years according to government policy?

No such confusion exists in the mind of a BUPA general manager. 'The NHS is a cost centre,' he explained, 'We are a profit centre. We are a business.' His task is to deliver a profit or he is fired. But he has to achieve these profits at the same time as achieving high scores in three surveys run annually by independent companies.

Staff, consultants and patients each have their own survey of about 80 questions on their satisfaction with the hospital. They are asked a wide range of questions in what the general manager described as 'a robust appraisal' of management and himself.

The survey's results are open to scrutiny. He arranges two hour workshops for management, 'so that they can understand the results fully and get the maximum out of it.' BUPA puts great emphasis on the surveys. 'It is very serious if the results of these surveys are weak,' explained the general manager, 'If I or any general manager continually receive satisfaction rates lower than is acceptable then I will not progress.' His performance is judged by the surveys. 'I am measured by this,' he explained, 'I am expected to show improvement year on year.' He also receives a financial incentive. 'If I achieve all my objectives I get a very handsome bonus in March. It pays for two really good holidays a year. I would be lying if I did not admit that this acts as a big incentive to me.'

The importance given to the surveys, their cost and the care with which they have been devised is BUPA's answer to a vexatious question: how to run a hospital that is both profitable (or in the NHS cost-constrained) yet of sufficient quality to satisfy its principal users, patients, staff and consultants. BUPA's solution is simple and certainly cheaper and more effective than that devised by Whitehall. It also ties the general manager directly to the well being of the patient.

The Government talks of patient empowerment. But real power – the power to affect a chief executive's career, never mind his holiday plans – is absent.

In contrast the NHS chief executive is instructed to achieve numerous, piecemeal targets that change all the time and which are devised by a third party, Whitehall. Good management means trying to meet short-term political targets designed by politicians for public consumption rather than the improvement of patient care. In other words it all sounds wonderful until you actually enter an NHS hospital. At the same time they are up against groups of staff with long traditions and well-established rights well aware that their chief executive will be moving on in a few years. In this situation it is very difficult for a chief executive to exert authority, make long-term plans or drive through reform – never mind safe-guarding the interests of his patients.

A director of BUPA who began his career on the fast track, NHS management course explained the difference. His former NHS chief executive refereed football matches as a hobby. 'That seemed to me very apt.' What a successful company needs is an outstanding striker who scores goals. 'What the NHS encourages is the referee who is balancing different interest groups. He is always chasing the game but never driving it.'

CHAPTER THREE

MIDDLE MANAGEMENT

A PORTER IN THE WEST COUNTRY had this to say on his hospital's middle management. 'We have 20 to 30 managers. Half of them don't know what they are doing. They hang around the coffee shop and get in my way when I am trying to push a patient through.' One of his patients, an entrepreneur, raised his head to stare, 'If I had that many managers,' he remarked to the porter, 'My company would be bankrupt.'

Middle management – defined here as those who have first-line managers or supervisors reporting to them and who report in turn to more senior managers at executive level – remains unaccountable to the public and untouched by the commercialism that transformed business in the 1980s. Roger Taylor, Research Director of Dr Foster, and who was otherwise optimistic about the Government's changes to the NHS, pointed to the poor quality of middle management in the NHS as the one factor to slow down the pace of reform.[28]

There are too many managers 'dead from the neck up,' said one chairman, 'and not enough,' said the chief executive of a North London hospital, 'making things happen'. He complained of too few experienced senior managers and poorly-trained middle managers. He wanted more and better managers and a job so attractive and well paid that he could recruit Oxbridge

---

[28]   Dr Foster is an independent organisation which collects and analyses information on the availability and quality of health services in the UK.

graduates. An auditor working for the Audit Commission with experience of both the public and private sector agreed that there was a shortage of good managers. In the last 10 years, 'The NHS has not attracted a high calibre of leadership.'

The NHS Plan calls for patient-centred care. This is a wake up call to NHS management. One they will take time to assimilate. Management are not used to thinking of the NHS as a patient service. Until now 'the bulk of managerial attention,' has been, as *Just Managing: power and culture in the NHS* put it, 'devoted to other groups of employees rather than towards patients.'[29] This was written in 1992 but is just if not more applicable today. Hospitals need good middle managers. But too much of what middle management does now is dictated by the centre rather than the needs of the patient.

Middle management see themselves as much put upon. Created in the first place to carry out political reform, they have suffered ever since from political whim. They find themselves caught between the demands of government for constant revolution and the medical professions which value tradition. Middle management is where the unreality of government speak meets the reality of too few staff and too many patients. It is an uncomfortable place to inhabit – especially for those with a clinical background. A manager in a north London hospital who deals with patient complaints described the worst aspect of his job, 'I can't tell the truth. I can't write your mother had poor care because we don't have enough nurses.' Another said, 'you are dealing with the same complaint over and over again. It's disguised in things like waiting times, discharge times but it all comes down to a lack of staff. It's very disheartening.'

Who exactly are these middle managers and what they do is a mystery even to the NHS. Three years ago health services chiefs

---

29   S Harrison, D J Hunter, G. Marnoch & C J Pollitt, *Just Managing: Power and Culture in the National Health Service*, Macmillan, 1992.

paid £500,000 to consultancy firms to tell them. They asked the Institute for Employment Studies to devise a 'workforce scoping exercise' to 'give us a picture of the management workforce.' Senior officials admitted they had no idea how many managers worked in the NHS or what were their roles. Nor did they know what skills management needed. One astounded doctor remarked, 'Can you imagine a firm like ICI or the Royal Bank of Scotland – or even your local McDonald's – not knowing how many managers it has? It's a joke. If the people at the top do not know how many managers there are and who's doing what, what hope is there?' An NHS official admitted that while they knew the number of chief executives and directors, 'it is the bit in the middle that is the problem.'[30]

"It is stopping us from hiring the nurses and consultants that we urgently need"
This 'bit in the middle' is expanding rapidly. Since Labour's election, from 1997 to September 2001, NHS management has increased by 22.6%. And figures released in June this year by the Department of Health show the numbers of managers in the NHS soared by three-and-a-half times the rate that nurse numbers rose between 2001 and 2002.[31]

Sir Nigel Crisp, the NHS chief executive is unrepentant. 'We do need good management in a system which spends £1 million every ten minutes,' he told the Public Administration Select Committee this year, 'We need to make sure we are actually controlling that properly.'

The increase in management numbers is a result of a shift in emphasis from the cost of health care to the quality of that care. In

---

[30]   *The Observer*, 6 August 2000.
[31]   The statistics define managers as staff with overall responsibility for budgets, staff or assets or who are accountable for significant areas of work. They do not include clinical managers, or junior clerical and administrative staff.

this the NHS is not unique. In the industrial democracies, it is now an article of faith that good science, proper information and appropriate monitoring will raise the quality of health care. In the US, this led to new government agencies devoted to improving quality standards and to private firms who promise to be able to separate good from bad physicians, hospitals and drugs. Amongst NHS management the watchwords are now performance evaluation, quality improvement, developing standards and monitoring compliance. Teams of outside people are constantly visiting hospitals to do just that in every sphere of hospital activity. No one is arguing against this. It is the way the NHS evaluates and monitors that is proving controversial.

Evaluation and monitoring requires people. In its 1995 yearbook, the Institute of Healthcare Managers listed 1,700 health service job descriptions. This year the figure has increased to an astonishing 5,529 and includes 41 different types of service manager and 50 different categories of project manager. They are all engaged in meeting Government targets, collecting data for the Department of Health, writing reports and checking their trust is compliant with various Government initiatives.[32] What they are not doing is looking after patients.

The non-executive director of a Three Star hospital in the West Country explained the process. 'When clinical governance came along, everyone thought great.' Then they realised they had to appoint a Clinical Governance Manager to make sure they were complying with Department of Health demands. But the Government provided no funds for this new manager or her secretary. Then they were told to put in place a partial booking system. Again everyone thought this was a good idea. But again the hospital received no money, 'Even though we had to appoint a general manager to organise appointments and bookings.'

---

[32]   *The Sunday Times*, 1 June 2003.

The new initiatives divert resources. The non-executive director explained, 'We are forced to make appointments that should be way down on our list of priorities.' When this happens ten times, the hospital finds itself with ten different initiatives, each of which requires a management department to implement them. 'it's a disaster.' She believed the initiatives to be, on the whole, a good idea, 'but we are having to use money from elsewhere to set them up. It is stopping us from hiring the nurses and consultants that we urgently need. We are so busy on these new initiatives that it takes money from the bread and butter work that we need to do.' So despite all the excellent ideas, 'care is going downhill and patients are not seeing any overall improvement.'

How the numbers grow is clear. The Burnley Health Care trust, for example, began its clinical audit in 1991 with two co-ordinators. It now has 6.9 whole-time equivalent staff and a budget of £170,000. In a recent survey of clinicians about half of the 35 questionnaires returned found its services satisfactory. 91% found its audit staff 'friendly and helpful.'

Chief executives are responsible and accountable for the quality of health care they provide in their hospital. This makes them, as one auditor said, 'very jumpy'. They are going to employ 'anyone and everyone to collect data' in order to reassure the Department of Health that someone is in place monitoring the latest initiative even if that information will do nothing more than, 'disappear up their own backside.' I emerged from one hospital board meeting befuddled by the sheer numbers of these initiatives and the complex procedures each required. In fact the whole board meeting had been taken up with compliance (apart from a passionate debate on staff parking). The chief executive agreed, 'When we hear of something going wrong elsewhere we say, "There but for the grace of God..." '

How much these new initiatives improve the patient's lot is difficult to assess. Health and Safety legislation, so powerful it can close down a hospital, does not, as one chief executive pointed out in surprise, include infection control. This is despite the fact that hospitals are filthy, that 5,000 deaths each year are attributable to hospital acquired infection and it is a substantial contributor to a further 15,000 deaths.

Risk Assessment, an NHS organisation set up to assess the risks to staff of doing their job, forced a woman with multiple sclerosis to sleep every night for 15 months in her wheelchair because nurses refused to put her in bed for fear of injuring their own backs. The NHS cancelled the nightly lifting service because the NHS Trust decided it was a 'highly dangerous task.' When the case came before the High Court, the judge found it 'extraordinary that a means could not be devised for lifting an 8½ stone woman once a day safely.' The woman had not slept properly for a year and had developed severe pressure sores. Her lawyer attacked as 'irrational' the trust's stance that the duty it owed its staff under health and safety laws 'trumps' its obligation to its patient.

But that is exactly what is happening in the NHS. In a world of limited resources, hospitals cannot afford seven clinical auditors, however 'friendly and helpful,' *and* seven nurses. It is one or the other. The Government has created the bizarre situation where hospitals take on managers to check and evaluate a service that is deteriorating because of their appointment. Which would the patient prefer? A hospital compliant with every government initiative? Or their ward staffed by a full quota of nurses? And would a hospital without staff shortages need so much monitoring?

A hospital board meeting discussed funding the newly set up PALS (Patient Advocacy and Liaison Service) another government initiative, to liaise with patients. Should they fund it for another year? The chief executive decided to go ahead because, 'we don't have the auxiliary nurses to chat to the patients and make sure they are alright. And our nurses are too busy.' In other words more nurses with the time to listen to patients would have done away with the need for PALS, its manager, two assistants and secretary not to mention its new office, freshly painted in lilac.

"It's a sausage machine!"

Political intervention, the emphasis on constant change and the lack of long-term planning has also meant an increase in management in the NHS. The social worker manager of one inner city hospital has almost trebled his team since 1997 from five hospital social workers to 13. He explained why this was necessary. In 1991 the Tomlinson Report pointed to a surplus of beds in inner London and urged the closure of 2,500 to 7,000 of them. The bed base in his hospital had shrunk from 2,000 to 450. But patient numbers have stayed the same. Whitehall had failed to forecast either capacity or its cost. They had not, for example, 'taken into account was an increase in the numbers of very elderly between 85 and 95 in the inner cities with complex medical needs.' He now lacked care homes to send them.

More than 63,000 care home beds for the elderly have gone since 1997 – the result, at least in part, of this Government's over-regulation. Many of the remaining care homes in his area did not have the facilities or qualified staff to look after the very elderly. He had just lost 25 beds with the closure of the cottage hospital. 'It's easier to get through the eye of a needle then to lay my hands on a continuing care bed.' He talked nostalgically of the convalescent homes on the East coast owned by the NHS but sold off in the 1980s. At the same time, he had to meet Government targets for hospital discharge. But as fast as he got them out, more came in, 'it's a sausage machine!' He had, with great ingenuity hit targets for the last 25 weeks. His reward? 'Government said reduce it by a further 25%.' He added bitterly, 'All I and my team are doing is trying to make up for the damage done by cutting bed capacity. It all comes down to that.'

A BUPA director who had been on the NHS fast track management scheme remarked on the average NHS manager. 'They are brilliant copers. But it's never more than a sticking-plaster mentality.'

"When are ministers going to calm down?"

All managers are subject to management fads; but NHS managers are more than most. Since its inception, the NHS has reflected every fashionable ideology. NHS management has had to absorb change at a pace that would defeat many other organisations. Legislation, circulars, guidelines, targets and demands for data flood the offices of the middle manager. Twenty years ago managers recalled 'Management by Objective' and 'Zero-Based Budgeting'. Now 'integrated care' and 'governance' has replaced 'core competencies' and 'outputs.' New management fads are promoted with the passion of a politician in a hurry. Rather than a coherent doctrine or long-term strategy, managers must deal with the 'ceaseless activity to grapple with the unacknowledged consequences of yesterday's mistakes.[33] Middle managers are at the mercy of politicians desiring major reform but not around long enough to pursue the incremental changes such reform requires.

The rapidity with which new management truths come and go gives the role of management in the NHS an air of illusion and instability. Is it possible to define management in the NHS when it changes every few years? Is it possible to judge what exactly makes a good manager?

Ceaseless activity from the politicians, ('when are ministers going to calm down?' asked one exasperated NHS manager at a conference) has a detrimental effect on everyone in the health service. In particular it hits those who must translate policy into action – the middle manager. They act as a buffer between the demands of senior managers for change and the ability and willingness of the clinical professions to cope with change. One recalled the usual response from nurses and doctors, 'Not more change' or 'Why should we improve quality just so our general manager can sail through her performance review?'

---

[33]   See C Hood, *The Art of the State*, Oxford University Press, 1998.

The constant re-organisations, I was told again and again, sap morale and breed cynicism. Since its inception 50 years ago, the NHS has been in a state of revolution. No NHS White Paper, for example, has ever been carried through in its entirety.[34] One consequence is that the NHS contains many young organisations, and others that have experienced major reconfigurations. The Quality Development manager of one London hospital complained of the 'constant priorities pouring down from the government. No one understands it. We are all doing it on the hoof.' Another said, 'We are in a constant state of start-up organisations.' It also makes a nonsense of the middle manager's efforts. You are hardly going to put your heart in a policy if you know from previous experience that in a few years time that policy will be side-lined, repudiated or just forgotten. One manager of PALS pointed out that each new initiative required a change of skills. 'The skills I acquired for fund-holding, for example, are now out of date. I can never build on my experience. I have to start each time from scratch.'

"We know that the numbers are wrong. We tell them that, but they are not interested"
Middle managers made the same complaint as top management. Too much time is taken up by the, 'obsessive desire for information' from the Department of Health. 'You're ruthlessly pursued for information,' said the waiting list manager of one hospital.

Hospital trusts are required to produce more than 600 pieces of information every month. The data collected by the Central Manchester and Manchester Children's University Hospitals NHS Trust for a study by the NHS Confederation, for example arrived in three large boxes and formed a tower more than six feet high.

Hospitals are taking on administrators just to collect information. NHS management journals are full of adverts for information analysts, service planners, user and patient access managers alongside programme facilitators, emergency service facilitators and

---

[34]   *Bristol Royal Infirmary Inquiry Report*, Summary.

shared care facilitators. Statistics have to be collected weekly and sometimes even daily on emergency admissions, day case surgery, trolley waits, bed occupancy rates, numbers of cancelled operations and so on. The NHS Confederation pointed out that even getting the required detailed information on just one of these statistics can take up to 200 pages.[35]

How much of this information is actually useful to managers? How much of it helps them run their hospital? The Audit Commission describes how managers develop 'parallel information systems: one to monitor and deliver service, and another to report on it.'[36] One example is the weekly 'Access Return'. This covers inpatient and outpatient waiting lists and times. It has to be submitted every Tuesday and relates to the previous Friday. One manager explained the problem. The information is required so soon that hardly any of the data has 'settled down', and is still full of errors and omissions. 'So we know that the numbers are wrong. We tell them that, but they are not interested. We would never use that data for our own decision making. Now, from October we will have to submit that return every day.'[37]

The Hospital Social Work Manager of a north London hospital said, 'So much onus is placed on demonstrating the precise nature of your activity that it eats into your time with your clients.' The Head of Treatment Management Systems in a hospital in the West Country agreed, 'I am so busy reporting that I do not have time to get on with any work.' Her trust had hired her to come up with 'creative solutions' to a number of problems. 'But I don't have time to see any of my ideas through.' Instead all her time was spent gathering information for the centre, 'we are being performance managed to death', and the work she wanted to do and which she believed would make a difference, 'gets short changed.'

---

[35]   *The Sunday Times,* 1 June 2003.
[36]   *Achieving the NHS Plan.*
[37]   Memorandum (PST 13) to the Select Committee on Public Administration submitted by the NHS Confederation.

Another manager complained that the Department of Health set deadlines 'which are absolutely ridiculous'. She is sending off figures every day and getting 'a barrage of questions' in return. She has to agree the information with a lot of people who in turn get fed up with her. One manager at a series of workshops held at the King's Fund saw everyday life in the NHS 'as a process of attrition. There was a sense of being up against it and not a lot of laughter.' The Hospital Social Worker manager remarked that the last person he had taken on went off with stress after 12 days. The two before that had left after nine and 12 months. 'This job used to be a cushy number, a career for life. Now we are on the front line.'

Another wondered, 'What do they do with all the information? I would love to know. The feedback is zilch which is disheartening. I don't mind doing the work but what I get back is minimal either in encouragement or approval. I can't even see the link between what we send them and the indicators they return to us.' Another remarked sadly, 'I don't know what the bigger picture is – I am trying to second guess what is the bigger picture. I guess nobody knows. It changes all the time.'

Information gathering does not come cheap. Salaries for these new managers can reach £60,000. Their appointment at the expense of front-line staff goes part of the way to explaining the discrepancy between spending on health care and the benefit to patients. Between 1999 and 2001 hospital funding increased by 21.5%, but the number of completed treatments rose by just 1.6%. 'Looking at the data, there is no discernible connection between the amount of money going into the NHS and the number of patients treated,' said John Appleby, chief economist of the King's Fund.[38]

The pressure to achieve targets is equally intense and the results as one consultant pointed out are 'frankly fraudulent'. A manager in a North London hospital said, 'Decent, otherwise

---

[38] *The Sunday Times*, 1 June 2003.

scrupulous people are pushed into conniving with the Government into hitting targets at the expense of patient care.'

There are numerous examples. Hospitals can offer appointments at short notice then restart waiting times if the patient cannot attend. This complies with Department of Health guidelines. It allows some trusts to achieve their targets. But it is no way to treat a patient. Cancelling high numbers of operations the afternoon before the due date means that the commitment to rearrange within 28 days does not apply. The manager meets the target but again this is little comfort to the patient.

It goes further than guidelines. The NHS Plan set a target that 90% of patients should wait less than four hours in casualty departments by the end of March 2003. The method of achieving this excellent target, however, was a disgrace and rendered it meaningless. First the Department of Health warned hospitals that waiting list times would be measured in a particular week in March. Management immediately made preparations. They asked doctors to work double shifts and cancelled routine operations. One consultant noted the effect in her hospital. First two of her junior doctors were requisitioned to work in A&E that week. Then she found managers uncharacteristically patrolling the wards in search of empty beds. Nurses often fail to report an empty bed in order to have fewer patients to look after. The managers were checking for themselves, 'So why don't you do that all the time?' demanded the doctor.

The ploy worked. The Government reported it had achieved its target: 92.7% of patients were seen within four hours. At least they were that week. Arrive in the same A&E Departments today and it is a different story. One hospital in North West England that met the target is now only seeing between 60% and 70% patients within four hours. On one day in April it dropped as low as 52%.[39]

---

39   *The Sunday Times*, 1 June 2003.

This dishonesty even extends to something as important as Commission for Health Improvement. CHI inspects hospitals every four years and is one of the corner-stones of the NHS Plan. Hospitals are given months or even a year's notice of a CHI inspection. They appoint a project co-ordinator to prepare the hospital for the audit (which will cost the hospital around £50,000). One such project co-ordinator explained, 'it's all very prepared and pre-planned.' She spends the time holding seminars for the staff to establish best practice and walking around the hospital to check compliance. After nine months of careful preparation, the auditors are finally allowed in. Their report is written and then, says the project co-ordinator, 'it is put on a shelf and forgotten about.' Three years later she returns, "sometimes they have carried through the recommendations, sometimes they haven't. It is not an ongoing audit. No one has gone back to check.' Such a stage-managed event may make the Government and the hospital look good. It is, however, hardly going to benefit the patient.

In contrast BUPA hospitals have three audits a year, one from the National Care Standards Commission which is announced in advance. The other two are organised by their own health care organisation. No warning is given. Inspectors arrive unannounced and will spend the day looking into every aspect of hospital activity. The report is then lodged with the National Care Standards Commission.

"You are forced to see patients as so many frozen peas"
Managers are the first to admit that too often they failed to do what a good manager should: question the value of existing activities, resource allocation or propose changes. Most of all they failed, as one auditor with the Audit Commission complained, to think of it as a patient service. 'If they did that everything would change. It's not just a lack of resources, it's poor management.'

Dr Gill Morgan of the NHS Confederation explained the problem. 'If you have centralist targets coming down from the top, the way you manage that at a local level is to be centralist yourself.' Or as one manager complained, 'you are forced to see patients as so many frozen peas.'

Constant nannying from the top induces a state of passivity. It is much safer just to do nothing. A manager pointed out that, 'One can go through a whole career without making a decision.' A bed manager in a north London hospital said, 'Decisions involve a degree of stress. Some people are not willing to get stressed out.' One manager of a flagship hospital in London recalled pulling letter after letter out of her predecessor's filing cabinet, each promising to 'discuss this further.' 'But,' she soon learnt, 'nothing had ever been followed up. He wrote all the right things but did nothing.' The head of Treatment Management systems in the West Country described meetings in a London hospital. Action points were listed and objectives set but, 'no one followed up afterwards to see if anything had been done – usually it had not.'

Clinical staff complained repeatedly of management stonewalling their ideas to improve patient care or increase efficiency. Years passed, meetings were held, opinions solicited but nothing happened. One young surgeon recalled being told to go away and write a business plan. 'I thought that was your job,' he complained. A consultant compared this to his experience in the private sector. There he made out his case on two sides of A4 paper, discussed it with the relevant teams then took it to management. They gave a decision within the week, put it out to tender and 'it happened immediately', – despite the fact that private hospitals are out to make a profit. It was not, he went on, just a question of money but 'a different, dynamic environment.'

A good manager will question activity and redesign processes. It can make a tremendous difference to patients. In the Leicester Royal Infirmary, for example, management counted the processes that happened to a patient from the time they entered with an ear, nose and throat problem to the time that they were treated. They counted 84 different interventions with the patient or their notes. They redesigned the system and cut it down to five interventions.

The young and energetic systems manager of a London teaching hospital explained her team's approach. Patients were waiting too long for ultrasound. First she analysed the problem. Was it a lack of staff or something else? She timed each procedure and worked out how long a list of patients should take to process. She discovered the lists sometimes started late because the doctors arrived late. 'It was very important not to jump to conclusions and rant at the doctors. Sometimes they were on call elsewhere.' The doctors never turned up on time because the nurses were always late setting up the clinic. Patients did not arrive punctually because they knew the clinic always started late. 'So we had to pull all that together.' Then she discovered too much time elapsed between each patient. Too often the radiographer had to stop and help the patient undress. So she employed people especially to undress patients and prepare them. 'This was much cheaper than employing a new radiographer.' It also made the patients happier. They are now undressed by people whose job it is to do so. 'They are much kinder than an radiographer who is impatient and cross because he thinks the delay will mean missing lunch.' These seemingly small changes have had a dramatic effect. The waiting time for an ultrasound has fallen from 13 weeks to under two weeks. 'We are now aiming for a walk in service.'

Then the surgeons in her hospital complained that patients were arriving late to theatre. This sometimes meant the last operation on the list got cancelled – a serious event for that patient. She discovered that otherwise fit, young people were waiting for a wheelchair to take them to theatre. Would they mind taking themselves, she asked. 'They ran downstairs.' Then she looked at another group of patients. They needed a porter and a trolley but did they need the nurse to accompany them to theatre? 'The porter was often delayed on the ward waiting for the nurse who was busy with something else.' Now that group could be collected by the porter on his own. Only a small number of patients needed a porter, a trolley and a nurse. 'It freed up the nurses and cost us nothing.'

Making things happen is the last thing many middle managers have time for. A senior non-executive said no one had a moment for 'a ground-up review' of previous plans and initiatives, to spot duplication and strip out what had ceased to be essential. Dr Gill Morgan, chief executive of the NHS Confederation believed, 'If you are spending all your time on the headlines, you will not be spending it on things which might be absolutely critical in your organisation.' People need, 'some protected time to think about what they really want to achieve for their patients.'

"We are all constantly surprised by the predictable"

Lack of good management systems is disastrous for the NHS. In January 2002 researchers at the Institute for Global Health tested the claim made by NHS Plan for 2000 that, 'The NHS is effective and efficient at meeting its goals. The NHS gets more and fairer health care for every pound invested than most other health systems.' It compared the NHS to Kaiser Permanente's California region because it is similar to the NHS in its organisation, its services and the amount it spends on each patient. The results did not reflect well on the NHS. Patients of Kaiser Permanente, the largest HMO in the US, had significantly better medical access than those on the NHS. For example in the NHS it took 13 weeks for 80% of patients referred to a specialist actually to see one. 80% of similar people in Kaiser Permanente's system saw a specialist within two weeks. 90% of Kaiser Permanente's patients who needed in patient treatment or surgery had such surgery within 13 weeks. Only 41% of NHS patients who needed such treatment received it after 13 weeks. Why was Permanente able to achieve such efficiencies? It places limits on hospitalisation. After adjusting for socio-economic factors, Kaiser Permanente had the equivalent of 327 acute bed days per 1,000,000 population. In contrast the NHS had 1000 acute bed days per 1,000,000 population, over three times as much.

MIDDLE MANAGEMENT

Hospital beds are the most expensive component of any health system. Inefficient use of beds leads to long waiting times. I came across constant scenes on the wards of beds blocked unnecessarily. A nurse did not report an empty bed to her bed manager because she was 'exhausted' and wanted a 'bit of a break'. One man discharged first thing in the morning had lain fully dressed on his bed until 7 p.m. that evening waiting for his prescription to be made up in the pharmacy.

Another woman wondered why the NHS had insisted she spend three nights in hospital before her operation. 'I thought there was meant to be a bed shortage. In a private hospital they operated on me within an hour of arrival.' An elderly lady begged the doctors not to send her home. She had no heating in the house and a 90 year old mother to care for. The consultant lost his temper. 'This happens again and again. We should have a service that swings into action even before she arrives. We have a discharge planning team, a liaison officer. Why aren't they here? Why are we surgeons having this discussion? She should leave on Friday. Instead she will go on Tuesday at the earliest.'

She is not the only one. 3,500 NHS beds are blocked each day by elderly people with nowhere to go. This costs the NHS, according to the Public Accounts Select Committee, £170 million a year and leads to the loss of 1.7 million days other patients could have spent on the ward.[40] Front-line staff were full of good ideas to ease bed-blocking. Often as the Systems Manager had discovered, it needed just a few minor adjustments. A sister pointed out that if one of her consultants visited his better patients first, instead of last, and another changed the time of his ward round, she could have patients discharged early in the evening rather than the next day. 'The NHS works on a fix-it basis,' she said, 'we are all constantly surprised by the predictable.' Her good idea had remained just that. Managers appeared uninterested or overwhelmed.

---

[40]   *The Daily Mail*, 17 September 2003.

This failure of management is an extravagance that the NHS can ill afford. If the NHS had Kaiser's acute bed day average, for example, it could save up to 40 million hospital days or £10 billion a year. These savings represent more than 17% of the NHS budget and could be spent on more and better paid staff, better equipment and facilities and improved information technology.

This lack of management systems permeates all the way down the NHS hospital. Two nurses in a hospital in the West country indignantly showed me their supply cupboard. Everything from the hospital suppliers 'cost a fortune'. They had only limited choice and were not allowed to shop around. They were also constantly running out, 'This week it's the disposable tissue holders', because management did not follow up orders. When managers ordered the wrong thing, 'they refuse to take responsibility.' The wrong gloves, for example had cost £12 to buy, £8 to return. 'The plastic funnel in the kitchen is £7!' While the price of toilet brushes so appalled the two nurses that 'we go down to Asda and get them for 69p.' Out of their own pockets, they bought hairspray and shaving foam for their patients. One held up a bar of soap. 'The suppliers only provide big bars. Each bar costs 70p and we can only use them once as each patient requires a new bar. Why can't we have small bars?'

Patients complain they often have to wait hours for a porter to take them for a scan. The porter manager of one hospital on the edge of London put it down to lack of resources. Their workload had trebled since 1997, pay was low and he was six porters short. But that was not what caused the delay as I discovered when I shadowed one of his porters.

Ray had been told to pick up a patient from A&E and get them X-rayed. First we had to find a wheelchair. There were none in the porters' bay. No system existed for tracking hospital property. 'There are never enough chairs,' said Ray gloomily. 'A&E bought eight last August. Now you try and find three!' On average, he reckoned, one got stolen every month. 'Pizza Hut is a good place to pick them up.' One was spotted in Clackton, another in Wood Green. Out with his family at weekends, 'I will suddenly shout out, "That's one of my chairs!"'

We set off in search of the elusive wheelchair. A porter, arriving back with a trolley, said he had seen one in Ottawa ward. This proved a good 10 minute walk away. We arrived to find it broken. 'Bits fall off all the time,' said Ray. Off we went again, passing another porter pushing an old lady. The two porters paused to exchange views of possible sightings of trolleys and wheelchairs rather like trackers discussing glimpses of a rare beast. The other porter thought he had seen a wheelchair the day before in Toronto ward. We turned around and walked this time for almost 15 minutes, having to cross outside twice. 'It's not a good job in the rain,' remarked Ray, 'and the patients don't like getting wet.' In Toronto ward where elderly stroke patients were forced to listen to the Rolling Stones blaring out from the nurses' station, no one had seen the wheelchair but they directed us to Montreal ward. Ten minutes later and by now feeling as if I really had traversed Canada's wastes we found a wheelchair pushed against a wall. A good hour after the request, we made it to the casualty department. The elderly patient looked exhausted. The nurse pursed her lips, 'Taking a tea break, I suppose?' she said. It would probably take the reader of this report no more than half an hour to sort out a system that would put an end to Ray's perambulations and the old lady's wait. No one has done it.

"Anyone who thinks they can manage a consultant is barking"

A key test of NHS management is how successfully they manage their doctors. Or as Rudolf Klein has written, 'how best to integrate experts into the policy machinery.'[41]

'Good managers work with doctors – but so few do,' said one auditor. The relationship is crucial, as both private hospitals here

---

[41]   R Klein, *The New Politics of the NHS*, Longman, 1995.

and HMOs in the States testified, to a successful, well-run and happy hospital. As a chief executive put it, 'things go wrong if you don't get it right.'

The relationship between management and consultants highlights the intractable problem at the heart of leadership in the NHS – the continuing and permanent excess of demand over supply for healthcare. This is a feature of a state health system that separates it from the private sector – the NHS does not have to advertise for customers. In fact it does the opposite – attracting fresh customers messes up budgets and overburdens staff. 'None of us want to attract more patients', said one consultant, 'we can't cope as it is.' Another said, 'The numbers just wear you down. I step out of the door into this sea of faces. I feel guilty just getting a glass of water.'

An ageing population, ever new and more expensive medicines and procedures means this situation can only get worse. Again and again, chief executives and management spoke of their concerns over capacity and the need to plan for more patients with more complex needs. It is almost impossible in an NHS, subject as it is to political pressure with the emphasis on good results now, to have the money or time to work out capacity and invest in the future.

In a state health service, the customer cannot choose how their money is spent. Managers make that choice for them. Their interpretation of providing patient care is to provide the greatest good for the greatest number in their community – the frozen pea solution. This brings them up against the consultant. His education and ethos is based on the right of his patient to the best possible care. He will fight any political objectives that put the interests of patients collectively over the good of his particular patient. This tension underpins much of the personal conflict, 'the adversarial relations' as the Bristol Royal Infirmary Inquiry put it, between managers and doctors which is doing so much to damage the NHS.

The antagonism runs deep. In every hospital I visited from the inner cities to the countryside managers and consultants rarely had a good word for one another.

Managers seemed flummoxed by their consultants' independence. As the Bristol Inquiry pointed out, consultants enjoy a job 'effectively' for life. They are extremely difficult to remove. 'They see themselves as largely autonomous, their duty owed to their patient, their sense of identification to their professional peer-group. To that extent, they do not see themselves as employees at all.' Or as one manager said, 'Anyone who thinks they can manage a consultant is barking. You have to have a relationship.' It is precisely that relationship that is missing in the NHS. As one chief executive said sadly, 'The system puts everyone at odds with each other.'

Managers complained that some consultants could display 'remarkable greed, interagency and trickery.' There is anecdotal evidence of consultants deliberately going slow on lists in order to encourage their patients to go private. A manager dismissed the consultants in her hospital as out of touch and under the impression, 'they are someone special.' Another pointed out, 'They might be brilliant surgeons but they are not trained in waiting lists and day to day stuff. They cancel operations at whim and do only what they fancy.' Yet another dismissed two of her consultants as 'a couple of Peter Pans. They are well into their forties now. It is bloody well time they grew up.' Explaining the lack of control over consultants in the Royal Bristol Infirmary, Dr Roylance, its chief executive, said he had not been in the business of 'herding cats'.

In any hospital drama on TV, the senior consultant is portrayed as a father figure, wise and all powerful. Rather like the concept of matron, this is wishful thinking on the part of the general public. Every consultant I spoke to from Three Star hospitals in the countryside to a Zero Star one in the city made the same complaint: the system does not work and their patients suffer. All put this down, in varying proportion, to bad management and lack of resources. As one consultant at a London teaching hospital said, 'It's just chaos – management don't take responsibility. They just don't care.' Ten years ago his work at the teaching hospital so absorbed him that the day spent on his private practice proved an irritating distraction. Now, 'It's a relief,' because, 'I can get things done properly.'

Many consultants felt their patients were subjected to poor nursing and, 'appalling physical circumstances,' as one said of his inner city hospital. They found themselves powerless to help. The consultant went on, 'I get letters from patients asking in astonishment what has happened to our once famous teaching hospital. I have very little power over that.' The influence he could exercise on behalf of his patients depended on personal contacts he had made in the hospital over 20 years. For a serious case, he might coax a scan for the next day, 'but I can't do that for everyone who needs it.' Another consultant in a rural hospital pointed out, 'I can't start treatment until I get a scan and a scan takes five weeks then another two to get the results. It's always a struggle.' The scanner closed at 5 p.m. and there appeared, 'no motivation', despite all the targets to keep it going all night, 'if that's what it takes.'

An Indian doctor from a zero rated hospital on the outskirts of London resorted to, 'flirting, battering my eyelashes and doing everything short of selling my body,' in order to cut the amount of time her patients waited for a CAT scan from over 11 days to under two. She was investigating one man with suspected brain tumour, 'What's that?' she asked pointing to pigmentation on his arm. 'Oh, I am on a waiting list for a biopsy for that,' he said cheerfully unaware he was already dying from secondary cancer. 'My patients are in pain and dying unnecessarily,' she said, 'and I can do nothing about it.'

Michael Gross, former NHS Consultant Neurologist at the Royal Surrey County Hospital in Guildford and short-listed twice for UK Hospital Doctor of the Year summed up the opinion of many, 'The real problem is the woefully inadequate treatment doled out to people with serious illnesses.'[42] By the time a patient has waited 10 days for a GP appointment, waited weeks to see a consultant, waited for a date for a scan, and then finally received a diagnoses, 'it could already be too late.' When he finally got to prescribe for the patient who had suffered their first epileptic fit or recurrent migraines, 'their quality of life had already deteriorated beyond belief.' Or as a consultant at a London hospital put it, 'On average the treatment in the NHS is crap. It is crap at every level. In the past we all knew we would get good care on the NHS. Not anymore. I have been a consultant in the NHS for the last 20 years but even I can't bully my way through the system. I don't trust it anymore. Five years ago I took out private medical insurance for my family. That's what I think of the NHS.'

The rise of the manager in the NHS has been at the expense of the consultants' power and prestige. The emphasis on budgets and quality control falls hardest on consultants. Their clinical judgements are constrained by budgeting and their professionalism by endless evaluations. 'We have been downgraded year after year,' complained one. Another said, 'Everything that made my work pleasurable has been taken away. Management constantly tell you, you are underachieving. It's about abuse and bullying tactics.' Michael Gross described his working conditions, a minuscule office shared with six other people. One telephone, no proper ventilation, no computer, not even enough chairs and one secretary he shared with three other staff members. A letter could take six weeks to turn around. 'We even had to empty our own rubbish bags.'[43]

Consultants resented being managed by people they did not respect. 'What about quality control on management?' asked one doctor. Management is not a 'profession' and managers do not have to reach an explicit standard to be qualified to practice. Nor do they have 150 years of powerful tradition or a scientific

---

42   *The Daily Mail*, 24 February 2002.
43   Ibid.

knowledge base equivalent to that of medicine. One consultant pointed out that he had four degrees and 'I am not unusual.' His manager is a former nurse. 'There is just no intellectual input. They are just not big enough people. Now I can talk to my chief executive on the same level. It makes a difference. I can't talk to my manager. It's like conversing with a child.'

Many consultants found the contrast in pay galling. A 'project' manager, as one consultant disdainfully said, 'whose training consists of the odd weekend course', can earn £50,000 a year. While a consultant with 14 years training and long experience is on £68,000 before the latest pay awards. One complained, 'I am 47 and I am earning less than my brother's secretary in the city.' He went on, 'my family have always been doctors but I told my niece she'd be better off becoming a vet.'

Many NHS managers have no experience of working outside the organisation. 'They would fail in a commercial environment,' said one consultant. Consultants who work in the private sector every week see the contrast starkly. One said that he, 'ignored' the management in his NHS hospital, 'they are so utterly hopeless.' They sent him lots of letters 'which I just put in the bin.' He described the private hospital where he worked which was run by one tenth of the managers, 'but they are very good. I speak to them frequently. I take them seriously. They are serious people.'

In the BUPA hospital I visited, the contrast is indeed compelling. In the NHS consultants are paid an annual salary irrespective of the number of patients they see. In the private sector they are paid by operation. The general manager of the BUPA said, 'I would never dream of micro-managing a consultant.' Instead he told his consultants, 'I can help you increase your earnings. It's up to you how you do it.' His consultants did not arrive late, nor did operations get cancelled. He found the power of the market far more effective than bureaucracy. 'If you have power financially, you don't have to use it.'

In a private hospital the consultants are customers as much as the patients. They can choose to work from a different hospital down the road. Their views in BUPA's annual questionnaire affects the general manager's bonus and ultimately his career. Just that morning a consultant had come in to complain that one of his patients was not being looked after properly. He had come directly to the general manager who had kept me waiting in order to sort it out. This is in complete contrast to the feeling of helplessness described by many consultants over the mistreatment of their NHS patients. Certainly one could not imagine them bothering the chief executive over the daily litany of lost patient records, late results and indifferent nursing – nor the chief executive putting everything aside to deal with the complaint. As one NHS consultant remarked, 'it takes four letters, at least, even to get a response from my chief executive. One year later nothing has still been done.'

This relationship is vital to the well being of the patient. The NHS Systems Manager of a London Teaching hospital showed what could be achieved. She worked with consultants to reduce rates of MRSA[44] and the average length of stay on her hospital's orthopaedic ward. She explained that the good idea is just the start, 'the difficulty is getting people to work together.' She put great emphasis on collecting data because 'doctors respond well to data. They respect evidence.' She gave her orthopaedic consultants 15 different graphs on patient throughput. She built them a computer module. They experimented with adding a bed here, taking one out there and seeing the result. Then she made a deal with the orthopaedic surgeons – control over their beds.

Only patients who had already been tested as MRSA negative were allowed onto that ward. Even if the ward had an empty bed and a patient needed that bed, they first had to be tested. This was

---

[44]   MRSA is the acronym for Methicillin Resistant *Staphylococcus aureus*, a bacterial infection increasingly found in British hospital patients. See Chapter 5.

vitally important to the consultants but, as the System's Manager admitted, 'a difficult concept for the managers to grasp.' They had targets to meet. 'How could we justify leaving a bed empty when beds are so precious in a hospital?' But the plan worked. Rates of MRSA fell not just among orthopaedic patients but overall. By reducing rates of MRSA they have reduced lengths of stay in the hospital as well. She said, 'Managers and doctors both want to improve patient care. We just come at it from a different angle; they, through individual patients, we, through system efficiencies. It all comes down to the same thing. You can't impose an idea on a doctor. You have to reassure them it is for the good of patients and not just to squeeze money out of the system.' It is no accident that she was one of the few managers I met who spoke of 'our consultants' with admiration and pride.

The reaction of the consultants is not unique. Many NHS staff would leap at the opportunity to do their job properly and to work in a well-organised and professional environment. Few are given the chance. Middle managers should be creating that environment. Instead they find their time taken up by the demands of the centre. Largely created by those demands in the first place, their priorities are to fulfil political targets rather than improve their hospital. In these circumstances it is not surprising that middle management is so ineffectual. Their failure affects nearly every sphere of hospital activity but, most of all, patient care.

CHAPTER FOUR

FRONT-LINE MANAGERS

ONE PORTER REMARKED on the nurses, 'Why do you need a degree to wipe bottoms?'

The Government recognises that delivering the NHS Plan will require, 'first-class leaders at all levels of the NHS.' In practice this is not happening. The further you move down the hierarchy of an NHS hospital, the more invisible management becomes. At the level of the patient, management is too often absent or ineffective. It is here that the crisis in NHS management is most acutely felt.

The patient exists in a power vacuum. Who is in charge of my health? Who is responsible and accountable for what? These are the questions any patient in a badly managed hospital will ask with increasing panic. Instead of the patient-centred service this Government promised, one woman noted in 'frustration, fear and fury,' when her daughter was hospitalised, are 'battalions of individuals employed to do their own tightly defined jobs and nothing more.' She feared without her intervention into her daughter's care, 'it could so easily go wrong, with potentially devastating effect.'[45]

No one person appears to have the authority to oversee all the elements of a patient's care, pull them together and take responsibility for that person's well-being. Whether you enjoy attentive nurses, a proper diet and clean wards is pot luck. As one patient remarked, 'After my last operation for a mastectomy I had

---

[45]   *The Times,* 26 November 2001.

no nursing. There was only one nurse on the ward. I could barely get to the lavatory on my own. My daughter had to bring in food, help me wash and comb my hair. The nurses never brushed my teeth once. This time I have been well taken care of.'

The Accident and Emergency manager

It starts even before arrival on the ward. Many patients complained their experience in A&E was as bad as the accident, illness or mugging which had brought them there in the first place. A publisher of glossy magazines found himself in an inner city A&E Department in the small hours. In one corner pimps rolled joints. In another a tramp was trying to commit suicide. 'It was only 10 streets away from where I live but it was another world. And very frightening.'

It is also violent. Drug addicts, people with knife and gun shot wounds arrive for treatment with friends and families. Fights erupt. A department that was busy but 'ticking along,' completely degenerates as doctors and nurses have to restore order. They also have to deal with the confused and the insane. Those on the fringes of society end up in hospital far more often than the middle classes. No one is turned away from A&E. Hospital is the last resort when all else fails. I came across one man lying in the admission's ward, all his belongings in four bin liner bags stacked up around his bed. He was alcoholic and diabetic. He beckoned me close. The night before, the nurse station had transformed into a cocktail bar and a blond nurse had served him a martini. He did not think he had imagined it. But could I check just to make sure? His landlord had thrown him out, his family had long since given up on him, social services had lost him but he still had a hospital bed.

In this frightening environment, patients complained that no one appeared to be in charge. No one was on their side. Junior doctors stared at computer screens. Nurses, either inexperienced or from agencies, were distracted or brusque. As the publisher commented, 'What this place needs is a good editor.' These are the managers to whom front-line staff report. Where are they and why are they not making their presence felt?

The forthright manager of one inner city casualty department was clear what stopped her. It was not the violence, the sheer number of patients, problems with her 80 nursing and clerical staff but the bureaucracy and the 'endless meetings'. An emergency would come in. She wanted to be on the shop floor, relieving staff and soothing relatives. Instead she would have to leave to attend, 'a bloody meeting about cleaning the bloody department.'

In any month, she managed just four or five days working, 'where patients and staff want me.' She spent only one fifth of her time with patients, 'it should be at least a half.' Instead she attended meetings on transportation, cleaners and upkeep. Each meeting required a member of staff from each department to attend and lasted at least an hour. She dismissed them as a waste of time. Rather than have to turn up, 'I should be able to say, "this is good, this is bad, get on with it."' A brisk, organised woman, she nonetheless admitted to feeling 'swamped by paper work.' A sudden crisis, 'it's the nature of A&E,' forced her to take paperwork home. 'If I was here until 7 p.m. or 8 p.m. every night, I could get it done. But I have a family and I refuse to do that.' She explained there was a lot of pressure at her level to stay late and even attend meetings that only began at 6 p.m. 'It's bloody ridiculous.'

It was also 'ridiculous' how much authority she lacked to get things done for her patients. The lack of authority cost her time. Cleaning and maintenance, 'terrible in this hospital' took up most of her energy. Her A&E department is open 24 hours a day and is used by 90,000 patients a year. 'Look around. You can see for yourself how grubby it gets.'

Before privatisation, A&E had a 'wonderful cleaner' who was loyal and accountable. But the new contractor reduced her wages and withdrew her holiday pay. The cleaner left. Now the department was cleaned by a Nigerian doing a computer degree.

He was a good man but paid 'peanuts' and was not interested in the job which is 'hardly surprising'. More importantly she had no say in his salary or his hours. If he slacked off, she could not reprimand him. She had to call the cleaning manager who was never around. When she did corner the cleaning manager, she felt forced, 'to shout and scream,' in order to get any reaction at all. Then, 'things will improve for a week. After that it slips again and we are back to where we started.' No one appeared interested in enforcing the terms of the contract. She went on, 'The company gets paid millions and millions to provide cleaning and maintenance – so why is the service so bad?' Just before my arrival she had been to the lavatory and found no lavatory rolls, 'Why should I be chasing up loo rolls? Yet that is what I have to do all the time. Because if I don't do it, no one else does and the patients complain.'

The manager of A&E had no say in the cleaning contract. She found herself forced to live with its terms – however inconvenient. The contractors clean up if someone vomits in the A&E department. However if a patient vomited in the waiting room, the cleaners refused to touch it because public spaces were not included in the original contract. The contractors define a waiting room as a public space. They also refuse to touch blood because that requires special training. She said in exasperation, 'The company is employed to offer a cleaning service. Why don't they train their staff to clean?' The week before a patient complained about a pool of blood in reception. The A&E manager explained, 'I usually mop up the blood but we had a trauma victim come in and I was with the parents. The patient in reception did not understand that I was busy.' In the end the receptionist cleaned it up. No one appeared to mind if she was trained or not.

Maintenance appeared to be another area over which the A&E manager had no control to the patients' detriment. It, too, took up a great deal of her time. She explained, 'What should I be doing this morning? A trauma victim came in. In order to free up the nurses to deal with the emergency, I should be caring for the relatives. Then there is a personality issue amongst my staff. That will take two or three hours to sort out. Those are vital things but what am I actually spending time doing? Chasing up loo rolls and dealing with the automatic doors to reception. They are stuck. Have you heard of an A&E department which you can't enter because the doors are stuck? Well, that is us. It is quite an issue when patients can't actually get in. But in order to get a member of maintenance staff here to fix them, it will take me a day of jumping through the hoops.' This is in marked contrast to BUPA hospitals where the head of maintenance reports directly to the chief executive and maintenance staff are working at a problem within the hour.

A week before, the resuscitation room had flooded. She jumped through the prescribed hoops but still no one came. Finally she evoked Health and Safety Regulations, threatened to close down the whole of Accident and Emergency and inform the chief executive. 'I should not have to do that.'

In the corridor of another A&E department an old lady was lying on a trolley. She had arrived at 10.30 the previous evening. It was now after lunch time. 'It's very hard on the bones,' she said, trying to smile, 'I wouldn't recommend it.' She had not been given anything to eat, 'and I haven't had a wash either. Of course they try their best, ' she added. A nurse had brought her a blanket and pillow but every time she turned over the blanket fell on the floor. The nurse had then provided her with a hook to pick it up, 'but I can't work it,' she said fretfully.

The A&E manager also finds herself powerless to protect her staff and patients against violent members of the public. A porter showed me the weapons recently taken from patients in a Zero Star rated hospital on the edge of London. Apart from all kinds of knives, including a butcher's boring knife, the collection boasted a beer opener stained with blood, a metal spoon sharpened to a point and aimed at a doctor's throat and a metal disc with razor edges which had been hurled at a nurse.

A young doctor back in London after working in a hospital in Los Angeles explained what happened when he called security staff to deal with a violent patient in his West London hospital. To his astonishment, they refused to touch the patient. They were afraid of being had up for assault. In Los Angeles police and County Sheriffs patrol hospitals and are trained to physically restrain and strap down violent patients.

The doctor pointed out the importance of this. Apart from the security of staff and other patients, 'we can't assess a patient until they are safe.' He went on, 'Here we can't send the patient home and we are not trained in restraint. It is a nightmare.'

Violence comes in many forms. I watched a small nurse in her twenties help a large, old woman into a wheelchair. Suddenly the old woman elbowed the nurse hard in the breast and stamped on her foot. An equally small and youthful, female doctor approached with a hypodermic needle, 'Get it in her,' yelped the nurse. The old woman made no sound but without a glance at the nurse belted her again. The doctor tried to inject her in the bottom. But the wheelchair was in the way and the old woman now showed an amazing agility, sliding her hips from side to side while still striking the nurse. It was like trying to dart a silent and malevolent rhinoceros. Finally the old woman collapsed into the chair and, with a grunt of satisfaction, watched the nurse limp away.

Modern matron

In an attempt to improve patient care and provide strong leadership, the Government has brought back matron. Before drawing up the NHS Plan, the Government took views from 152,000 members of the public and 58,000 NHS staff on how to improve the service. The single most requested item was the return of matron, a strong clinical leader with clear authority at ward level. Someone in charge of getting the basics right, 'without getting bogged down in bureaucracy.' 2,000 of these easily identifiable 'modern matrons' with their own uniform and a 'modern, enhanced set of responsibilities' have been introduced after an absence of 30 years. (In the private sector matron has remained alive and well.) Stephen Thornton, then chief executive of the NHS Confederation, saw the creation of a modern matron as 'essentially an investment in management and leadership in the NHS.'

The NHS's rejection of an authority figure in the 1970s articulated a more general social trend of that era. That trend appears undiminished today. Many nursing staff and unions appear uncomfortable with the idea and perplexed by its popularity dismissing it as 'sexist,' and 'playing to the *Daily Mail*' reader. It raised a romantic 'good old days' when hospitals were ruled by a rod of iron and matron checked for every speck of dust.

Nursing organisations have been quick to take up the grit of the modern matron and refashion it into something softer and more acceptable. The authority figure becomes, according to Sarah Mullally, Chief Nursing Officer, 'professionally and emotionally supportive of staff' while allowing nurses to 'take control of the environment.' At the same time, reassures the Royal College of Nursing website, they will exude, 'a professional calm' while engaged in 'emotional labour.' Unfortunately emotional labour is not quite what patients had in mind when they asked for the return of matron.

The public may confuse modern matron who is in charge of three or four wards with the sister who is in charge of one. However they are quite clear what they want: someone with authority to oversee their care. BUPA still has matron who is a powerful figure, second only to the chief executive.

Thirty years ago, matron's role was undisputed. It was to run her hospital and wards. She knew all her patients, her nurses, her cleaners and the porters. She had authority over every one of them. A porter in a rural hospital in the West country recalled that in the 1970s, 'If matron saw my hair grow below my peak cap, she fined me 20p which went into the charity box.' A nurse from the same era described how her matron would measure her skirt every morning before starting work. It could be no shorter than 15 inches from her ankle. The same porter said that matron had a say about who to hire and fire. 'She'd announce, "So and so is out" and that was it.' Now, he went on, everything has to go through a disciplinary procedure. 'It's very rare anyone gets fired. You certainly can't dismiss a porter on the spot.'

The majority of a matron's time was spent walking the wards. Her authority extended into very aspect of her patients' care. No detail was too small. One porter recalled a matron coming across a broken chair in the corridor, 'What's it doing here. Get a carpenter and get it fixed.' Now, he went on 'the waste is awful. I see 200 new computers just go out of doors. As for a chair, a slight rip and it's out too.'

Sister's role has also changed. It took six to seven years experience to make a ward sister. Now it can be as little as three years. She checked her patients received suitable food and made sure that they ate it. Now she has to call a dietician. She saw herself as the patient's advocate. Her opinion was sought and valued by the consultant on his ward round. It also meant if something went wrong or was not done, she took responsibility. The blame stopped with her.

The role of matron and of sister has changed out of all recognition. Thirty years ago a large number of patients in hospital were convalescing or dying. Now patients are in for a shorter time but are much sicker. Modern matrons and sisters are also now responsible for their own budgets. 'I spend hours in finance meetings,' complained one. She has to put in a business plan for her ward every year and plan the number of nurses she needs and of what skill mix. She needs to fill in audits and assessments. What she has less and less time for, is being on the ward, checking her patients and supervising her junior nurses.

An Irish sister of 17 years' experience in a hospital in north London admitted she had a mountain of paper work, 'lots of questionnaires and pilot schemes. I think too many. You can hardly breathe without some kind of policy' that she simply ignored. 'I should spend one day a week on it but you can't be away from patients to have a ward function well. You have to maintain a high presence on the ward. I am double checking everything because that's my job. I tell my nurses we have lives at stake, like it or lump it.'

She saw no point in promotion even though it meant she lost out financially. Her next grade would take her up to modern matron with overall responsibility for four or five wards. But promotion took her away from her patients. 'I enjoy my work. I like being with patients and nurses.'

"I do like to have a chat if there is a problem"

I met several of these new matrons and shadowed one who I will call Daphne for half a day in an inner city, London hospital. As the sister predicted, we spent very little time with patients. It was a quick walk through the wards with the occasional stop for a chat. Unlike the matron of 40 years ago, Daphne did not know any of her patients or what they were in for; nor did they know her.

In the men's surgical ward all but one of the men had been injured committing a crime. 'Last week we had someone with a bullet wound,' the sister told us afterwards, 'Sometimes we have a policeman on duty. Of course the other patients don't like that.' The only man not to have committed a crime lay neatly curled up on top of the sheets in pyjamas. At the foot of the bed a diminutive nurse sat on a stool reading *OK!* magazine. He was from a secure lunatic asylum. The nurse was there to guard him. I pointed out she was very small. 'But she can read his mood and prevent him doing something,' said Daphne.

On the female ward I stopped in horror in front of an old lady in a blue bed jacket. Her face was a mass of bruises. I assumed she had been brutally mugged. Daphne looked embarrassed. A wrong prescription from her GP had left the old lady dizzy. She had tripped over and broken her hip. The bruises were from falling out of her hospital bed. An old man next to her, who had somehow found himself on the woman's ward, piped up that he had already complained just that morning, 'People are falling out of bed all night long. Thump, thump, thump. They do it so much they wake me up.' I asked Daphne why the beds lacked the cot sides available in private hospitals. 'We believe physical restraint is inappropriate to our patient's dignity,' reproved Daphne.

The 'big part' of Daphne's day, she admitted, was spent in meetings. She named 10 off the top of her head: a clinical board meeting every three months; a food and cleansing meeting; a Blue Team meeting; a Critical Care Delivery Group every six weeks; a meeting with all the heads of surgical wards every month and a subsequent meeting with ward managers to pass on that information; an audit of Risk Assessment every six weeks to see what had gone wrong and how it could be improved; a glucose monitor review group; the meeting of a Flexibility Group in order to improve retention and recruitment of staff... 'And that's not all,' she finished.

She was proud to attend and rated the meetings highly, 'I have been nominated for all these meetings. They are a big part of the day but necessary. You do need to be involved. People are including me in the decision-making process. They are taking decisions at these meetings that will affect my job!'

Modern matrons are supposed to have the authority to get the basics right for patients. But in the emotionally supportive NHS culture how easy is it to exercise authority at this level on behalf of the patient? The contrast with the all powerful matron figure of 30 years ago is stark.

A patient in one of Daphne's wards had been waiting all morning for a porter to take her for a scan. The porter had failed to appear. In the corridor, Daphne bumped into one. 'It's stressful for the patient and frustrating for the nurses,' she explained. The porter shrugged, unmoved. His workload had tripled that day and three men were off sick. There was nothing he could do, he said and moved off.

The matron watched him go undecided if even this mild reproof had been too forceful. Eventually, as if seeking confirmation, she said, 'Well, I am glad I mentioned it. I do like to have a chat if there is a problem.' I asked if there was any occasion when she could sack a porter or at least issue a reprimand. She looked shocked, 'Oh no, we can't get rid of porters if they are no good. We send them on a training course.' Meanwhile the patient continued to wait.

It was the same for the food. An Indian patient had ordered a vegetarian meal. Twice the meal had come up incorrect. Finally the patient had given up and not eaten anything at all. Daphne took it up with the kitchen, 'a lot of ward sisters would not have bothered but I do.' Her power, however, seemed limited to complaining. She went on, 'things might improve for a month but then it all slips back again.'

She had worked briefly in the private sector, 'Patients expected to be waited on hand and food,' she said in surprise.

Daphne was clear on her role. She saw it as passive and sympathetic, 'I am here as a listening ear for everyone.' She believed she had power, 'but you can't use it willy-nilly or you loose it. You can't just go and whine. You have to negotiate.' This view was echoed by other modern matrons. Back in the 1950s and 1960s, 'it was much more hierarchical,' explained one, 'now it's more a case of working with people to achieve goals. You can't go around saying: "Do this" or "Go and do that now". It doesn't work like that any more.'[46]

This meant Daphne saw her role towards patients as less champion more pacifier. Patients, she said with an air of surprise, still demanded to see matron when something had gone wrong. She found a 'softly, softly,' approach the most effective. 'I am here to defuse anger because there is so much anger amongst our patients.'

---

[46] *The Evening Standard*, 15 September 2003.

I witnessed an example as I was leaving. Two Turkish men were shouting at the nurse. Their mother's operation had been cancelled at the last moment. Daphne moved in to placate them in her element as 'the listening ear.' The nurse sighed, 'The sons are all concern now but once their mother's had the operation, they'll expect her to carry her own bag out of here – and cook dinner once they are home.'

There are no doubt many modern matrons who are making a tremendous difference to the patients in their care. I met sisters who through sheer personality, hard work and devotion ran exceptional wards. But Daphne's experience shows how difficult it is to exert authority on the patient's behalf in today's NHS. Both the system and the culture connive against it.

Nurses

A crucial part of a matron's time was managing her nurses and training junior staff.

Modern matrons and sisters admitted that meetings and administration cut into this vital task. The problem was exacerbated by a shortage of nurses, in particular a shortage of experienced nurses (those on D and E grades), and a reliance on agency nurses. Care was noticeably better in the rural hospital in the West country. They had few staff vacancies, had rarely employed an agency nurse and their D and E grade nurses had worked in the hospital for 10 years or longer. Many matrons and sisters pointed to chronic understaffing and nurses too young and inexperienced for the responsibility forced upon them. As one modern matron said, 'There is nothing I can do to help. It is very stressful for them.' This lack of management has had a disastrous effect on patient care.

A nurse consultant who prepares hospitals for audits gave an example of the scene she comes across every day in the NHS. She walked into a ward where a second year nurse was taking care of six patients unsupervised by a senior nurse. The sister was not in evidence. An old man wearing an oxygen mask was sitting in bed staring disconsolately at a wash bowl. Next to the wash bowl lay his breakfast, uneaten and besides that, an overflowing sputum pot. A full bottle of urine dangled beneath the bed. The nurse had abandoned him with the wash bowl, 'to do what he could'. The nurse consultant said, 'It was a revolting sight.' No one had taught the nurse first to clear everything away, remove the urine bottle and then present the bowl of water.

No one had taught her the purpose of nursing; to do for the sick what they cannot do for themselves.

The training of nurses has promoted them further and further away from the interests of their patients. In the late 1980s, nursing turned itself into an academic profession. Nurses, desiring increased status and greater parity with doctors, sought to transform their training into a graduate profession. The result is 'a frigging mess' according to a member of the King's Fund.

Nursing became 'embedded in a power struggle' against the doctors, the NHS and even the patients 'should patients ask nurses to do anything that undermined their status' states Julia Magnet.[47] One senior staff nurse at a hospital in the West country who teaches at the local university pointed out that the academic status of the qualification meant, 'there has to be a lot of theory.'

The Florence Nightingale school of nursing and midwifery at King's College London gives a flavour of the sort of things nurses are now expected to learn. 'The social context of health and healthcare, which considers the relevance of sociology and health policy to healthcare.' Integral to the course is, 'exploration of key sociological issues, which influence healthcare such as poverty, gender, social class, ethnicity, and race.'[48]

A staff nurse who had recently qualified and was working in a London A&E department complained her training had not prepared her at all. There was too much theory, social policy and

---

[47]   *Prospect*, December 2002.
[48]   Ibid.

communication skills – and not enough practical. In 18 months of study she had spent only one and a half hours learning how to take blood pressure and a patient's temperature. On the other hand a whole afternoon had been devoted to poverty in Russia. 'They don't prepare you for the things that matter,' said the staff nurse. Instead she learnt how to approach a patient and what mannerisms to adopt, 'Well, if you don't know that, why are you becoming a nurse?' she wondered. Or as the Irish sister of 17 years put it, 'No, I have never felt the lack of studying sociology. Kindness and common sense go a long way.'

The staff nurse was astonished to discover how little anatomy or physiology her course contained. Anxious that her grasp of these essential subjects were, 'not as good as they could be,' she approached her tutors. But they took a more relaxed view. She soon discovered her ignorance did not matter. Her first exam, tackled after 18 months, was multiple choice. Her final exam, at the end of two and a half years, allowed her to answer three out of six questions and so avoid revealing her ignorance. She managed to qualify with only a vague knowledge of the bodies soon to be in her charge.

Instead her tutors set her assignments on social issues and ethics – including patient rights. That a patient might have a right to a person properly qualified in their care did not seem to have occurred to her teachers. She said, 'Theoretically you could go through the whole three years without any one asking you about bed sores.'

Her training left her unprepared for her new role. She recalled vividly putting on her uniform for the first time and pinning on her badge. She looked at herself in the mirror with a sense of disbelief. 'You are expected to cope with situations which you know you just can't. There is no one to ask. Or they are too busy or they don't know because they are agency nurses.' Another nurse recalled the shock of her first days on the ward with phone calls coming in from everywhere and acutely ill patients.

In one 10 minute period she had to arrange transportation for a patient, give morphine to a man screaming for pain relief and see to another in a side room, dangerously short of breath. 'I was on my own. I did not know which way to run, which was the most important. I remember thinking, 'Shit, I just want to get out of here.' She went on, 'I learnt more in the first three months on the job than three years at college.'

The Irish sister had scant respect for new nurses, 'They picture themselves at a computer or with a doctor on his rounds. They are horrified to discover that 90% of their time is doing things for the patient.' They think it is enough to offer a bedpan to a patient once every four hours. 'I tell those nurses, if the patient asks for a bedpan 40 times in a shift then they need it. I see nurses walk past a patient ignoring his distress. I will not have on my ward a patient apologising because he needs to ask for care. We are dealing here with sick and vulnerable people many of whom are dying. I aim to see them die in dignity and comfort and that their relatives will have good memories of their last few weeks.'

The Irish sister had a very different training. She learnt practical skills side by side with what she was studying in the class room. She practised washing a patient and making beds. Every three months she did a three hour exam in the morning followed by a two hour one in the afternoon. 'You went through things over and over again,' she recalled, 'if you failed an exam, you had one chance to repeat it, then out. You also had to go through every task observed by a nurse until you were ticked off on it.'

A former matron recalled being watched and criticised 'and woe betide if you got anything wrong' while learning to wash a patient, feed them, put on a dressing and make them comfortable. 'No one learns how to make a patient comfortable anymore,' she said sadly. Rather like the concept of hot milky drinks, which as a junior nurse she offered patients every night at 8 p.m., it got jettisoned in favour of social policies.

Once on the ward, 'a nurse took you under her wing to show you the ropes,' recalled the Irish sister. Nowadays overseeing and training newly qualified nurses can get overlooked. One staff nurse said the atmosphere on her ward was very unfriendly, 'you screw up your courage to ask someone to show you a procedure and they give you a withering look.' A sister explained when a nurse asks for help, 'you have to set aside half an hour to show them how to do it. If you don't give them the time they will make a mistake. But we don't have the time.'

"She's not my patient"

Thirty years ago it was very different. In those days of task-centred care, the newly qualified nurse knew exactly what was expected of her. In one morning she might be asked to polish all the bedpans, or give each of the 17 patients on the ward an up-bath. As a senior nurse she dressed all wounds on the ward. In the mid 1970s task-centred care changed to client-centred care. Each nurse was allocated a group of patients for whom they did everything. 'All it did,' she recalled, 'was create a mountain of paper work.' Nurses had to asses their patients then plan their care and all this had to be written down. It was fine if there was enough staff. But if a nurse had to cover for a colleague, she suddenly had 10 patients whom she knew nothing about. The former matron recalled a relation asking for a bedpan for her mother, 'She's not my patient,' reproved the nurse.

The irony is that nurses thought that by making their qualifications more academic, they would gain the respect of consultants. This does not seem to have happened. Nearly every consultant I interviewed complained that the standards of nursing were, as one put it, 'dangerously low.' He went on, 'it's very frustrating to see our patients treated to such poor standards of care.' A consultant anaesthetist at a London teaching hospital complained of patients arriving for operations with bed sores. On ward rounds he frequently helped patients to eat. 'The catering staff slam the food down. No one bothers. Spooning food into a patient is just too demeaning for professional nurses, it seems,' he added, 'I always thought nurses were meant to care for patients. I might be wrong. I may have missed the plot somewhere.'

Another described the difficulty of visiting one of his patients. Every patient is meant to have their name above the bed. But in some hospitals they refuse to display the name 'in case it infringes your autonomy.' So the consultant finds himself wandering around trying to find his patient. 'There never seems to be anyone in charge who knows anything.' Then trying to find the patient's nurse. Then trying to find the patient's notes. 'I don't often strike lucky with all three.' Then he has to translate the nurses' diagnoses. 'They refuse to use hierarchical, male dominated medical terms. So they will not say the patient is unconscious. No, the patient has to have "an altered state of awareness".'

The voluntary service co-ordinator of one hospital where he had worked for many years passed a room. An elderly lady called urgently, 'Please take me to the toilet. I have been pushing and pushing the button but no one will come.' He pointed out that only a nurse could take her and went to find one. Three were clustered about the nurses station listening to Radio 1 and dipping into a box of chocolates. He explained the situation. 'Can't you hear the patient calling?' 'Oh she's always calling,' they said without moving. 'Never mind if she wants to go, she wants to go.' He went back and found the old lady face down on the floor. He returned to the nurses, 'You had better come now,' he said, 'I think she's dead.' He added, 'That has happened more than once.'

One woman noted that her daughter's nurses were 'friendly enough' but 'they were not paid to take responsibility, so they do not. They may all need degrees now but, with the plethora of catering staff and orderlies, their role seems limited.' She thought it would be reassuring if at the start of every shift they came around, introduced themselves and announced that for the next few hours patients were in their care. 'Instead, they go diligently about their form-filling.'[49]

Many patients had stories of neglect. One woman suffering from a placenta praevia found herself abandoned in a side-room. No one came. No one checked her blood pressure or temperature. Her catheter was left in for three days. The toilets were all blocked up. Finally her cousin, herself a gynaecologist, arrived and was so appalled she had a show-down with the nursing staff. 'I would have had better treatment in the Third World,' remarked the woman.

Many told of unexpected kindness and good nursing. One woman recalled, 'The older ones are better. The younger ones are quick to tell you, "That's not my job" or "That's not my patient."' 'An older nurse had taken her down to the theatre for her operation and kissed her, 'it was so comforting and sweet. It made a big difference to me.' But whether patients received a kiss or a reproof for 'whinging' as did one man after a traumatic road accident, seemed entirely a matter of chance.

The attitude of the nurses is of enormous importance to a patient who is helpless and totally dependent. It is bad enough being ill and in pain. To be abandoned or treated unkindly is almost insupportable. Traditionally, the sister attended the ward round with the consultant. Sisters saw their job as taking the patient's side and putting the patient's point of view. They had after all taken care of the patient over the last 24 hours. The loss of their authority means the loss not just of patient care but also a patient's advocate.

A member of the King's Fund questioned the whole basis of 'life-long learning in the NHS'. She said, 'it's an uphill battle to continue their training if they are no good in the first place.' Education is expensive, raises expectations and does not solve the lack of staff. Nursing is mainly done by young women and there is a constant turnover of them. 'We need more nurses on D and E

---

49   *The Times*, 26 November 2001.

grade.' But the only way to gain promotion or an increase in salary, up until recently, is to move into management. This takes nurses and auxiliary nurses away from the patient and the practical care at which they might excel.

Sir Stanley Kalms remarked, 'People say nurses are angels. Well, nurses are employees who do nursing.' Like every other employee they need managing.

The modern matron lacks the tools to manage her nurses. One former matron, now a nurse consultant in audit work, pointed out the difficulty of disciplining a nurse for incompetence. First the busy matron or sister has to notice. Most are too occupied or away from the ward to take it in. Then even if she does, discipline in the no-blame culture of the NHS is a 'long-winded process'. The emphasis is on being, 'nice' and making sure it is no one's fault.

She continued, 'You can't bawl them out or they'll sue you for harassment.' Instead 'in a nice soft voice, you have to ask if that was the way she had been taught? Did she consider it appropriate care?' Modern management is meant to 'nurture' its employees. The errant nurse is offered training, supervision and given another chance. This can go on for a year. 'In the meantime,' said the former matron, 'patients are going through her hands and suffering.' Most matrons or ward managers take the easier option and promote the incompetent, 'to get them out of your hair.'

Even if the nurse is disciplined, the modern matron faces a further difficulty. Who will replace her? A bad nurse is better than no nurse. Low pay and a shortages of nurses insulates the profession from the normal disciplines of working life. Trusts around the country are struggling to find the staff they need for present work loads let alone those needed to take forward planned government activity. To replace those retiring or leaving, to fill vacant posts and to meet Government targets, Greater Manchester, for example, needs 2,071 new nurses. Recruitment from overseas and new trainees will mean 1,455 nurses by 2005-6. This leaves a shortfall of 616. The trust is experimenting with a cadet scheme.

Nurses enter the profession to care for people. Their training and lack of supervision on the wards robs them of the means to show their compassion. Those that do manage to give good care succeed despite the system not because of it. A male modern matron with 15 years experience in the NHS summed up a view I heard from nearly every medical person I interviewed including many nurses themselves, 'I would not trust my dog let alone my mother to many of them.'

The failure of management around the patient is evident in a number of different areas. Patients, for example, complained about the food. It was inappropriate for their age or illness (elderly people can be flummoxed by pizza), it was just bad or did not arrive. 'My family bring me sandwiches,' said one old lady, 'most of our friends do.' Another commented, 'I just took one look at it and I said no.' One woman had not eaten for 48 hours. 'They did offer me a tea cake which had been in the fridge for months. I had to throw it away.' Nurses seemed indifferent or helpless.

The *NHS Magazine* states that 40% of adults are suffering from malnutrition on hospital wards. Many elderly patients arrive malnourished but studies show their condition deteriorates in hospital. Malnutrition results in 'substantial' morbidity and mortality, complicates illness and delays recovery as well as reducing wound healing and increasing the risk of infection. The King's Fund estimates this costs the NHS £226 million a year. The fact that so many of our elderly are actually going hungry on our wards, unnoticed, is an appalling indictment of the NHS and the management of those wards.

'Essence of Care', distributed by the Department of Health, is an indication that even it is concerned about what is happening on NHS wards. 'Essence of Care' describes best and worst practice for patient care from bed sores to feeding and patient notes to incontinence. The book categorises levels of care beginning with, 'deliberately negative and offensive behaviour and attitude.' These basics are what nurses 30 years ago learnt as a matter of course.

These basics were nursing. Now the Department of Health has to regulate something as fundamental to the sick person as privacy and dignity. As a member of the King's Fund said, 'What state must nursing be in that the NHS should have to put around this?'

The foreword by Sarah Mullally, Chief Nursing Officer, makes grim reading. 'Essence of Care' she writes focuses on those 'core and essential aspects of care' that matter to patients 'quite rightly' yet which rarely attract the attention they should during the 'quality improvement process.' You cannot help but wonder at a 'quality improvement process' that fails to notice bed sores or malnutrition. They are described 'as the softer aspects of care' crucial 'to the quality of the carer/patient experience.' She suggests a weekly tea party where carers and patients can 'express concerns'. Here then is our modern culture of caring. Bed sores and malnutrition alongside tea parties and a happy experience for all concerned.

The lack of management around the patient is due to matron's loss of power and the shift from the practical to the academic in nurse training. These reflect cultural preferences both in the NHS and in society as a whole. But they have taken precedence over patient care.

The Government is not addressing these issues. To do so, it would need to give hospitals the power to pay nurses a reasonable wage. It would need to face down vested interests and give modern matrons the power to hire, fire and reward staff.

I met many dedicated sisters and nurses. But dedication is not enough. There is only so much difference an individual can make against a system that fails to support them. The focus of health care on the patient has been lost. The impact on the patient is devastating.

CHAPTER FIVE

INFECTION IN THE NHS HOSPITAL

AT EVERY LEVEL, NHS management lacks the authority to get things done and to improve patient care. It is particularly weak at dealing with issues that need fundamental system redesign and cross-departmental work involving large numbers of clinicians and managers. There are many examples of this: the failure to run a credible appointment system, the failure to look after patients' notes satisfactorily, hopeless IT systems and, perhaps most immediately threatening to patients' health, Hospital Acquired Infection (HAI). Dirty hospitals, high on the list of almost every patient's complaint, is a direct result of a management system in crises.

Hospital Acquired Infection affects 300,000 people a year. 5,000 die of it and it contributes to the death of a further 15,000. It costs the NHS more than £1 billion a year and looses 3.6 million bed days. British hospitals have higher rates of infections than Greece. The danger of contracting the bugs here is more than 15 times higher than the next safest countries which include Iceland, Sweden and the Netherlands. Many strains are so virulent that entire wards and operating theatres have to be shut down and cleaned.

The most notorious infection is MRSA. There is only one antibiotic strong enough to treat it MRSA, Vancomycin and even that is loosing its power against the most virulent forms. Since the early 1990s the number of MRSA infections in hospitals has soared from 1% to 45%. The symptoms of MRSA infection are boils, wounds that will not heal, fever and acute pain. This leads to blood poisoning and the devastation of internal organs and bones.

The main means of catching HAI is through the dirty hands of hospital carers. Fewer than 5% wash their hands between touching patients as they are meant to. Professor Hugh Pennington, an infection control expert at Aberdeen University, warned of the crises facing patients unless staff start taking hygiene seriously, 'I have investigated slaughterhouses cleaner than some hospitals', he said. Retired GP Roger Arthur whose wife died of MRSA believes the full extent of MRSA is being covered up as doctors are reluctant to record it as a cause of death. He said, 'The true statistics would cause panic.'[50]

In the past, hospitals took cleaning seriously. Florence Nightingale had reduced the fatality rate of the wounded soldiers in the Crimea from 40% to just 5% just by imposing basic standards of hygiene and sanitation. Forty years ago matron checked levels of cleanliness every morning. One consultant remembered that his hospital set aside a ward just for cleaning staff to learn how to clean. Cleaners were valued members of the team and worked with the medical staff. All cleaning, for example, was done before ward dressing in order to let the dust settle before exposing wounds to the air.

Things are different now. Dr Leyla Sanai, a former consultant anaesthetist for the Western Infirmary, Glasgow wrote recently about her experiences as a patient. Despite her job, she was, she admitted 'utterly ignorant' of the real conditions on an NHS ward. Hospital managers keep consultants – and visiting politicians – in the dark by ensuring that main corridors and ward entrances are kept clean, thus creating the illusion that standards of hygiene are being maintained.

Then she became a patient herself. In the toilets she found 'a pile of faecally-soiled paper underwear, a blood-stained theatre gown, used dressing or a filthy toilet bowel.' Not once in her three week stay did she see the cleaner bring a mop into the bath room.

---

50   *The Daily Mail*, 16 September 2002.

She noticed some pubic hair on the floor of the shower. 'So I kicked it away with my toe and saw it settle in the corner of the room.' Three weeks later when she left the ward, it was still there. On one occasion she was moved into a room on the acute surgical ward just as the previous patient was being wheeled out. There was no attempt to clean the room between their stays. Another time a nurse took the thermometer from under the arm of one patient and, without wiping it, 'thrust it under my arm,' then placed it back in its container, again without cleaning it. She was not surprised when she caught MRSA.

Dr Roger Arthur, a retired GP, was shocked to see when he visited his wife in hospital, dead flowers in vases, sweet papers, old bits of Elastoplast and the tops of disposable syringes behind the bed. He said, 'The condition of the ward did not change at all from the first day I went in to visit my wife. It was disgusting and dirty.' He was told that her operation had been successful. Within hours of returning home she collapsed. Tests confirmed she had MRSA. She died from blood poisoning four days later.

A consultant anaesthetist working in a Zero Star hospital on the outer edges of London described the state of her theatre. Blood is splashed everywhere and patients are coming in and out for operations. 'We don't get time to clean between patients. But they do in private hospitals and the turnover is just as fast.' In the past it was someone's job, for example, to wash all theatre staffs' shoes every day. 'Here no one does it. The surgeon's shoes are caked with old blood. I wash my own.' In the private hospitals in which she also worked, the theatres are closed every six months and cleaned thoroughly. Bacteria swabs are taken before opening again. 'We have never done this in my NHS hospital.' She had tried to interest management but they had been 'very obstructive.' A year later she was still waiting to hear. Infection rates after hip operations were high. She claimed any patient staying in her hospital longer than a week was in danger of catching MRSA, 'I would not come here if I was sick and it is my local hospital.'

"That's not my job"

The cleaning of wards is no longer under the control of medical staff. It is now the job of the cleaning manager and outside contract cleaners. Staff complained the problem lay in management's ignorance about cleaning and their inability to negotiate a contract. Dr Leyla Sanai used to watch the cleaner arrive with a grimy mop and 'a bucket containing nothing more than a puddle of black water.' The cleaner had to get through six wards of 40 patients in a few hours which gave her only a few minutes in each room. 'Consequently she would just empty the bin, half-heartedly clean out the sink and then run the ragged mop over the visible areas. Not once did I see her change the fetid water in her bucket, add detergent to it, or clean under any beds.'[51]

One Filipina who has been a cleaner for many years in the NHS explained, 'No one tells the cleaner to change their water when it gets dirty. If you don't stipulate in the contract that the water should be changed four times when you wash this floor, they won't do it.' They do not know to wash the mop and stand it up after it has been cleaned. If the floor must be scrubbed and not just mopped that too has to go into the contract.

One community psychiatric nurse suddenly discovered that her manager had not thought to include clinical waste in the cleaning contract. The cleaner simply shrugged and said, 'That's not my job.' When she persisted she was told to ask his boss. He said the cleaner did not have time and besides it was not in the original contract. 'It drives me daft,' she complained. A Filipina nurse was shocked that her NHS hospital had no cleaners during the night. 'In the Philippines we have lots of cleaners round the clock. Here I have to clean everything up myself after 6 p.m.'

The NHS Plan promises the new modern matron will be given the authority to resolve issues 'such as poor cleanliness.' Front-line managers dismissed the idea of having any authority over their

---

51   *The Daily Mail*, 24 January 2003.

cleaners. Hospital management awards the contract to a cleaning company. 'What are we meant to do?' asked one modern matron, 'renegotiate a million pound cleaning contract all on our own?'

The hospitals I visited appeared powerless to do anything about MRSA. This was true at every level of hospital management. It illustrates the lack of effective management to push through change and exert authority – even for something so essential to patient care.

"You've got to have eyes in the back of yourhead with these girls"

The issue was raised at one hospital board meeting. A consultant explained how he had provided A&E with text books to which staff could refer. Then he noticed that junior doctors were 'sticking their fingers into ulcers' looking up something then moving onto another patient or the computer key board. He suggested removing all books and covering the keyboards with cling film. This suggestion was warmly greeted. It was much cheaper than the other option up for debate – 24 hour cleaning at a cost of £60,000 a year. The consultant then admitted, 'I don't get stroppy with staff if they do not wash their hands.'

'I do,' replied another doctor.

'But you are a surgeon,' pointed out the first, 'and I am just a gentle physician.'

Stroppiness is not seen as a virtue in the NHS. Yet how can patients be cared for properly without it? The chief executive sighed, 'Thirty years ago we had matron to uphold cleanliness. Now we are reintroducing matrons.' He did not sound hopeful.

Nor should he be. A few days later in the same hospital I was shadowing Daphne, one of the new matrons. She was telling me of the importance of a clean environment. The nurse manager from Infection Control arrived to discuss where to place the dispensers of alcoholic rubs. This was to solve the problem of how to make nurses wash their hands in between patients. At the moment few could be bothered or had the time. The sinks were outside each ward. It meant walking to them between patients. Another disincentive was the Hand Rub itself – stinging and drying to use.

The two women discussed where to place the dispenser of alcoholic rubs in order to catch the eye of the busy nurse. We tried the wall behind the patient. But would the nurses bother to turn around and reach up? The two women thought not. We then moved to the foot of the bed. Could a dispenser be hung there? The two women shook their heads again. They felt sure the nurses would not feel like bending down. Not even for patients' safety, I asked. The two women sighed. Would the threat of the sack or a fine make the nurses more amenable, I went on. Both women looked horrified, 'That's harassment,' they said firmly. Daphne added, 'Anyway we would have to sack all our nurses and where would we get replacements?'

Finally, Daphne suggested hanging the dispenser at either end of the ward. This was a piece of typical NHS fudge. We all knew the nurses would never use them. But the dispensers, so prominently displayed, would reassure senior management and inspection teams. They would not, of course, do the patients much good.

We were standing in front of a side room containing a patient with MRSA. Earlier Daphne had shown me the apron and glove dispenser at the entrance of the room. Every nurse had to put these on before touching the patient, then remove them before leaving the room. Suddenly I noticed a nurse walk in, see to the patient then depart. She had not touched the dispenser. This was done in front of matron and the infection control manager. Neither appeared to notice. In astonishment, I interrupted the two woman. Had I misunderstood? It appeared not. Daphne tut-tutted, 'You've got to have eyes in the back of your head with these girls,' she said. The infection control manager nodded sympathetically, 'Doctors are far worse,' she added. The two women turned back to the problem of the dispenser. There was no question of a reprimand.

The high levels of HAI are an indictment of NHS management. They have failed at every level to exert authority and pull together the groups involved for the benefit of the patient. One porter summed up the vacuum that now exists. When he arrived on a ward 30 years ago, sister immediately approached him. 'What are you doing here?' she questioned. When he mentioned a patient's name, she knew who it was and where they were going. 'Now I just wander around,' he went on, 'before matron had control over me. Now it is down to 20 or 30 managers who don't know what they are doing.' NHS staff may not like the idea of working in an organisation where they could be reprimanded and sacked. But it would revolutionise patient care not to mention raise morale amongst those many staff who want to work in a well run and professional atmosphere.

CHAPTER SIX

CONCLUSIONS

THE PROBLEMS OF NHS MANAGEMENT are bound up with the problems of the institution itself. The NHS is a vast, bureaucratic organisation, top heavy with administrators and is expensive and 'strikingly inefficient.'[52] Reform is piecemeal and has failed because it has not engaged with the basic premises of the NHS. It was 'designed' to be state-owned, centrally planned, centrally financed and centrally run.

Aneurin Bevan admitted its ideological basis in 1958 during the tenth anniversary celebration debate of the NHS in the House of Commons when he said, 'The redistributive aspect of the scheme was one which attracted me almost as much as the therapeutical.'[53] Sir William Beveridge, the architect of the NHS promised that his proposals would take the country 'half way to Moscow.'[54] Fifty years on, Russia and China are shedding their monolithic state industries. We still have the NHS.

Every incoming Government promises to cut back bureaucracy in the NHS. Then it increases management to carry out its initiatives. While the NHS is controlled at the centre, management numbers expand at the expense of front-line staff. This is the nature of a state bureaucracy. They are self-perpetuating, take on their own life and are, as even Richard Titmuss, Professor of Social

---

52   S Lawlor, *Second Opinion? Moving the NHS Monopoly to a Mixed System,* Politeia, 2001.
53   Quoted by R Klein, op. c.it.
54   Quoted by N Timmins, op. cit.

Administration at the London School of Economics and a passionate advocate of the British Welfare State, admitted, 'independent or impervious to the public they are presumed to serve.'[55]

The series of paradoxes that defines the NHS also defines NHS management. Public funding versus professional integrity, constant revolution versus disheartened and cynical staff, the demands of the centre versus the needs of the hospital and ambitious and often conflicting goals versus unadmitted choices and trade-offs; all these and more hobble the NHS manager.

At every level, NHS managers struggle against a system that will not be managed. They lack the necessary data, the authority and, in too many cases the ability and training to question existing activity, pull together the variety of different constituents in a hospital and push through policy. Their experience can be summed up by the following quotation:[56]

> We tend to meet any new situation by reorganising and a wonderful method it can be for creating the illusion of progress while producing confusion, inefficiency and demoralisation.

This was originally written by Caius Petronius nearly a thousand years ago. How many more years must we wait while politicians try to change the unchangeable?

In our attachment to the principle of the NHS we have allowed a vast bureaucracy to replicate itself at the expense of our health. The dedication and perseverance of NHS staff ensures that some patients get good treatment, some of the time. But it is in spite of, not because of, the system. As a country we can no longer afford any top down changes. The history of the NHS shows they work fitfully and have unintended side effects. The NHS must be decoupled from political interference and power transferred from

---

55   Quoted in S Lawlor, op. cit.
56   This quotation is taken from N Timmins, op. cit.

the bureaucracy to the patient. Until there is real competition between providers and some surplus capacity within the system, patients cannot exercise choice. And it is patient choice that will do more than any government policy to force good practice up through the management hierarchy. In the meanwhile we have allowed authority and accountability to absent themselves where they should be all important.

Recommendations

Every developed country is struggling with the cost of its health system. The head of one of the largest and most successful HMOs in the US talked about 'the illusion of efficiency.' Even the most efficient management cannot make up for the cost of an ageing population, chronic illness and ever new and more expensive procedures and drugs. In this situation the NHS boasts one advantage over its rivals. It is a superb instrument for rationing. Moreover it still commands such loyalty and affection that people believe in its mystique even as they die on some waiting list.

NHS managers have to manage a business where demand will always exceed supply. Any increase in quality only attracts more customers. In the private sector, managers use pricing in order to restrict supply. NHS managers cannot adjust prices, cannot invest in more capacity and do not control one of the most important components of their costs: wages.

Any recommendations have to be set against this background:

1. Patient choice – or as probably, the threat of patient choice – will force good practice up through the management hierarchy. The Government's proposals for foundation hospitals are therefore a welcome first step on a much longer road.

2. Chief executives must have the ability to fix salaries and hire, fire and reward staff.

3. Political management of the NHS has failed and will continue to fail. Money must follow the patient throughout the system.

4. A robust system of audit, accountable to parliament and with strong powers – including the power to close a hospital down – should be introduced. Auditors should make random inspections without notice.

5. The audit system should operate no more than five or six targets. This will allow chief executives to look at the overall performance of their hospitals rather than to fixate on bits of systems.

6. Satisfaction levels of patients, staff and consultants should be surveyed on an annual basis. This, together with financial performance and the numbers of patients treated satisfactorily, should be the basis on which the chief executive is to be judged.

7. Replace targets on waiting times with simple computer-based information available to the public. In Denmark hospitals publish their waiting times on the internet.

SOME RECENT PUBLICATIONS

WELCOME TO THE ASYLUM £10.00
Harriet Sergeant

The Government has lost control of immigration. Britain is now seen as the softest touch in Europe. Government failure corrupts and criminalises. And immigrants, who are dependent on criminal gangs to claim asylum, are the first to suffer. The breakdown in the system is responsible for a man starving to death on the landing of small house in Streatham, a 10 year old working for a few pounds a week, sometimes just for food, in a factory in Wembley and a child imprisoned and forced into sex day after day in central London. Can the next generation of refugees survive all the indignities of immigration – the gangs, the slave labour, enforced prostitution, a sink estate in Glasgow – and go on, as their predecessors did, to dazzle us with their achievements?

A brilliant exposition… Sergeant's work should be studied by all politicians –
Stephen Glover, *The Daily Mail*

…an engrossing new report which shows in chilling detail the extent to which this Government has lost control of immigration –
Christopher Hudson, *The Evening Standard*

RESUSCITATING THE NHS: a consultant's view £7.50
Maurice Slevin

The NHS is imploding. The huge increases in NHS spending will fail to produce the desired results unless the way the money is used is changed radically. The author – one of Britain's top cancer consultants – demonstrates that far too much of the new money has been, and will continue to be, wasted on a proliferating bureaucracy. Two reforms are essential: the balance of power and control in the NHS must be taken from the bureaucracy and given to patients; and the number of administrators in the NHS must be substantially reduced, thereby releasing funds to substantially increase the number and pay of nurses and allied professions.

…a report that will send shockwaves throughout Whitehall – Daily Mail

The pamphlet highlights the difficulty Tony Blair faces in delivering on his promises to transform the NHS with an extra £40 billion of public spending over five years – Financial Times

NO SYSTEM TO ABUSE £7.50

Harriet Sergeant

The NHS is being exploited. It is being taken advantage of by people from other countries who have no entitlement to our system of free health care. This is not the fault of the individuals concerned, but a systemic failure at the heart of the National Health Service. The problems are threefold. Firstly, the system is open to abuse. To the determined health tourist, it is relatively easy to get free health care. Secondly, the number of people arriving in this country who have a legal entitltement to free health care is also growing, and putting increasing pressure on the NHS. Thirdly, the great majority of immigrants – whether legal or not – are coming from countries where diseases such as TB, Hepatitis B and HIV are all endemic. In the absence of any system of control, the Department of Health is unfair on NHS staff, on genuine asylum seekers and on the ordinary citizen.

"Harriet Sergeant's explosive report on the abuse of the NHS by asylum seekers and illegal immigrants suggests Britain has taken leave of its senses" – Daily Mail

BETTER HEALTHCARE FOR ALL £7.50

Norman Blackwell and Daniel Kruger

Blackwell and Kruger argue that only by giving control of spending to patients, and control of delivery to professionals will we have the level of healthcare which we all want. The authors recommend liberalising both the supply of healthcare (by making hospitals and doctors independent) and the demand for healthcare (by giving all those who wish to opt out of the NHS an 'NHS Credit').

An important and illuminating pamphlet... The right has been criticised for failing to engage with the debate over public services... the CPS pamphlet goes a long way to addressing that criticism – Peter Oborne, *Sunday Business*

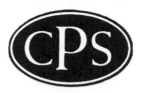

BECOME AN ASSOCIATE MEMBER OF
THE CENTRE FOR POLICY STUDIES

The Centre for Policy Studies runs an Associate Membership Scheme which is available from a minimum subscription of £55.00 per year (or £50.00 if paid by bankers' order). Associates receive all publications (of which there at least 15 in any 12 month period) and (whenever possible) reduced fees for conferences held by the Centre.

We also welcome donors who are prepared to subscribe additional amounts to help to support our ongoing policy work.

For more details, please write or telephone to:
The Secretary
Centre for Policy Studies
57 Tufton Street, London SW1P 3QL
Tel: 020 7222 4488   Fax: 020 7222 4388
e-mail: mail@cps.org.uk   Website: www.cps.org.uk